What people are

Meeting the Melissae

Meeting the Melissae is a marvellous invitation that celebrates our sacred bee and human history together. Elizabeth is a fantastic writer. The stories are deeply personal, richly joyful and viscerally challenging. Those illustrious qualities also make them relatable and enfolding. My favorite parts are how vividly her words carried me into lush surroundings and floral scents my nose recognized. These are stories I want to hear!
Jacqueline Freeman, Author of *Song of Increase*

The Melissae have been a subject of enchantment and deep study for me for many years. Their stories are enchanting, and their archaeological evidence engaging. Elizabeth's interpretations will delight and engage any reader, and make them fall hopelessly in love with the bee.
Andrew Gough, Historian and TV Presenter

Elizabeth Ashley gathers her encyclopaedic knowledge of Melissa Medicine to reveal the bee priestess as its energetic practitioner. *Meeting the Melissae*, through metaphor and myth, will introduce you to the ancient priestesses that served the Goddess Demeter as oracles and soul midwives. Ashley will then dance you into the fertile hive of history with her musings and correlations to unveil the Eleusinian Mysteries, where you will extract your own golden honey of wisdom and revelation.
Thea Summer Deer, D.S.P.S., Herbalist ~ Educator ~ Author of *Wisdom of the Plant Devas: Herbal Medicine for a New Earth*

Now more than ever, it is imperative that we protect bees and their relationship to the plants, and all biodiversity including human beings. *Meeting the Melissae* does more than highlight the deeply rooted ancient mythology and sacred relevance of Melissae – or bees. It carries a strong message for their preservation. This beekeeper's holistic approach captures their biology, highly advanced caste and communication systems, pollination techniques, and the many challenges they are facing. Her profound love for, and deep connection to the bees and other pollinators transcends even the mortal. An offering as sweet as nectar that offers many rewards for bringing us closer to this invaluable fragile species.

Dr. Kelly Ablard, CEO Airmid Institute

This book is a pot of honey, slowly dripped into my open mouth. It is nectar to my soul. This treasure trove weaves together the puzzle pieces of the Goddess Path across the Pantheons and timelines across Mother Earth. Deeply affirming and honouring. This book is well researched with documented facts together with personal gnosis that leads the reader through a rich honey pot of different textures, thickness and flavours. I am delighted to review this book by Liz. What has been lost is being reclaimed and re-membered. Thank you, thank you, thank you.

Angie Twydall, Sacred Bee Priestess, Creatrix of the Bee Oracle Deck, founder of Sanctuary of Sophia, Director of Temple of Avalon, Ceremonial Priestess at Glastonbury Goddess Conference, Womb Trauma Therapist and Teacher

Meeting the Melissae has all of the essential ingredients that the honey tongued will want to devour bud by bud.

Chronicling the proper dance of bees across ancient civilizations, while acquainting the reader with the bee priestesses and goddesses in a harmonious dance of alchemy.

A sacred experience, that will touch each reader differently. A journey that I will recommend over and over again, so that multitudes can experience the sweetness of each page.

Elizabeth Ashley is literally the bee's knees, and her writing is like a portal into the sacred teachings of the Melissae. Her words, like honey, were liquid sunshine for my soul.
Amanda Bjorvik, Melissa Bee Priestess

This book is a gift! Elizabeth is a brilliant weaver of words. I've truly enjoyed being swept away into this divinely feminine world of magic and mystery.
Mindy Sue Bell, Folk Herbalist and Intuitive

As a lover of bees, mythology and archetypes I thoroughly enjoyed Elizabeth's amazing *Meeting the Melissae*. It is a deep dive into the sacred feminine archetypes – human and beyond human – rites and lore related to bees and Melissae, their priestesses.
To me this book provides long-needed answers about the sacredness and symbolism of bees, as well as the Melissae, and many other mythologies that form the hidden underlying anatomy of our collective psyche. It is an urgent, much-needed book to help us reconnect to Nature and to ourselves.
Florian Birkmayer MD, Holistic Psychiatrist, AromaGnosis.com

This book is a gem... a fascinating glimpse into the intriguing world of the MELISSAE, an ancient and shamanic lineage of Bee priestesses linked to the goddess, Demeter.
Elizabeth Ashley leads us into a living world of ritual, sound, and scent, which will delight anyone with an interest in plants and essential oils but also their links with mythology and history. Each chapter reveals secrets and mysteries, and the realisation that the wise Melissae along with the Bees still have much to teach and inspire us... I urge you to read this book, as I did, on a summer's afternoon, amidst the dreamy sound of bees and the sweet smell of Lemon Balm. I can promise, you won't be disappointed.
Felicity Warner, Founder of Soul Midwives and Author of *Sacred Oils: Working with 20 Precious Oils to Heal Spirit and Soul*

I feel like I've been waiting for this book.

Ultimately, *Meeting the Melissae* brings the profound, but tauntingly incomplete knowledge of academic history into the re-emerging presence of the Bee Priestess.

As a devotee of spiritual practices tied to the honeybee, I have devoured academic sources on ancient beekeeping, and I have wrapped myself in the mythologies and modern devotionals of the complex deities who claim the bee as symbol. *Meeting the Melissae* is a new, approachable, and profound source of academic and spiritual information, and it will grace my nightstand for years to come.

Journeying through Elizabeth Ashley's discoveries felt like a mutual remembering of a long forgotten sisterhood. So much felt so very familiar. The rites of Eleusis – as researched and dreamed by the author – felt familiar. Finding yourself inside of a story is why so many of us love to read about the ancients. We imagine what it might have been like. Finding yourself *remembering* into a story is something else entirely. There's more going on here than just well-informed historical speculation. This is, let us call it, Kleiomancy at its best.

Speaking of the Melissae's Eleusis, I found deities there that I've come to know quite well. My experiences with Dionysus and Persephone tell me that they have been represented faithfully here, and I find myself encouraged to perhaps meet some new archetypes. The relationships that exist between the deities of Eleusis are complex and oftentimes disturbing. *Meeting the Melissae* handles these mythologies with fairness and respect, focusing primarily on the priestesses who served their imperfect Gods and Goddesses through their spiritual community.

I've never experienced a book which so respectfully avoids telling me what to DO or what to BELIEVE, but which so inspires me to follow my own intuitions and dreamings.

Anyone with an interest in the role of the priestess – ancient or modern, in the bee – especially as a symbol of the Chthonic, or in the mysterious rites of Eleusis, will find something here.
Jen Marie, Devotional Beekeeper, Rahibe of The College of the Melissae, Drinker of Wine, Eater of Pomegranate

Elizabeth Ashley weaves together incredibly readable Melittology (that's "bee science" for those not in the know) with inspiring anthropology of the priestesses, aromatherapy wisdom and fascinating renditions of mythology. Her writing is fun while at the same time studious and intelligent. Her book has deepened my knowledge immeasurably and brought forth many "ah-ha" moments both intellectually and in my shamanic practice.
Bee medicine has been very prominent this year and with society in such a precarious place it's no wonder that a metaphor of community care that functions so flawlessly has so much to teach us.
I highly recommend Elizabeth's book; in fact, I already have, to a number of people.
Ruth Cato, Shamanic Practitioner

Meeting the Melissae not only appeals to the practically & historically curious, but also weaves ley lines of routes thrumming & buzzing with destinations of goddesses and gods. They are returning to waggle dance the trajectory of the sun, to where the sweetest, most potent information, stories & knowings lay. *Meeting the Melissae* is informative, stokes curiosity & makes the most of the hive's propolis to ensure the anecdote of life with bee balm past & present is sealed.
I wish you a book of a prolific Queen whose daughters & sons dance & sing in celebration & sharing of the nourishing pollen & nectar that exists within the pages.
Darci Faulkner, Owner of The Shamanic Bee Healing Centre, Devon

Meeting the Melissae: The Ancient Greek Bee Priestesses of Demeter is a gorgeous and enchanted offering. With historical references, beekeeping knowledge, plant wisdom and sacred inspiration, Elizabeth sets the scene for what it means to be a powerful Bee Priestess. This book comes from a place of pure love. It's deeply inspiring and I enjoyed every word!
Kimberly Vincent, Bee Priestess, Bee Keeper, and Humble Spiritual Seeker on the Path

Beautifully written and encaptivating. A must-read for every woman, to get back to her roots and feel the strength from generation to generation. Deeply researched and full of information. An insight to the start of religions and influences which we see up to this very day. Who would have imagined that most rituals and ways of life were inspired and learnt from Bees. What Bees did naturally, humans copied as a way of life! The mention of my homeland, Malta, made it even more special. A book which needs to be read over and over again, one which will instigate the reader to live as close to nature as possible where everything makes so much sense!
Lorraine Spiteri ADipCT (VTCT-UK), Complementary Therapist, Reflexologist specialising in the treatment of pain

This fascinating insight into the world of bees and the Melissae takes the reader on a journey exploring the role of the priestess in different cultures and times as well as talking about the unique and extraordinary operation and life cycle of the hive. My long-held interest into bee spirituality has been rekindled by reading this book and has inspired me to investigate further.
Jenny Mawsley, Teacher

Elizabeth Ashley offers powerful insights into the extraordinary lineages of bee wisdom teachings and their unique emergence in ancient Greek civilizations. Ashley's personal testimonies, combined with her soulful, and thought-provoking deep dive, into the origins, belief systems, ritual practices, and medicinal functions of the apis mellifera, take us into the complex psychic universe of the mighty bee, and Her connection to the archetypal feminine in the time of the Melissae. Elizabeth Ashley invites us all to sit deeply with the bee, as entry into the ancient language that links its evolution to our human identity. Her mosaic of research presents us with a poignant call to remember the Melissae as emissaries of our responsibility to consciously hold and nourish the sacred hoop of our artful design within the constellation of our world's cosmic hive.

Desiree Mwalimu-Banks, Priestess, Interdisciplinary Artist, Educator

Meeting the Melissae

The Ancient Greek Bee Priestesses
of Demeter

Meeting the Melissae

The Ancient Greek Bee Priestesses of Demeter

Elizabeth Ashley

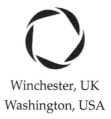

Winchester, UK
Washington, USA

JOHN HUNT PUBLISHING

First published by O-Books, 2023
O-Books is an imprint of John Hunt Publishing Ltd., 3 East St., Alresford,
Hampshire SO24 9EE, UK
office@jhpbooks.com
www.johnhuntpublishing.com
www.o-books.com

For distributor details and how to order please visit the 'Ordering' section on our website.

ISBN: 978 1 80341 249 8
978 1 80341 250 4 (ebook)
Library of Congress Control Number: 2022938607

A CIP catalogue record for this book is available from the British Library.

Design: Lapiz Digital Services

UK: Printed and bound by CPI Group (UK) Ltd, Croydon, CR0 4YY
Printed in North America by CPI GPS partners

The author of this book does not dispense medical advice or
prescribe the use of any technique as a form of treatment for
physical, emotional, or medical problems without the advice of a
physician, either directly or indirectly. The intent of the author
is only to offer information of a general nature to help you in
your quest for emotional and spiritual well-being. In the event
you use any of the information in this book for yourself, which is
your constitutional right, the author and the publisher assume no
responsibility for your actions.

We operate a distinctive and ethical publishing philosophy in
all areas of our business, from our global network of authors to
production and worldwide distribution.

Contents

No tree can grow to Heaven unless its roots reach down to Hell.
– Carl Jung

For my beloved husband, The Strong Silent One, for my gorgeous sons, Andrew and Dexter, and for my mom and my sisters. You are my rocks.

For Ariella Daly of Honey Bee Wild and Jennifer Naylor of Lomah, a Land of Milk and Honey. May your hives swell in size and cast many swarms.

For my Dreaming Hive and fellow Magdalena Melissae.

For Deby Atterby, with humblest thanks for always having a fellow bee in your back pocket. For Angie McKay, for your never ending faith in this book, and for my Uncle Dave, with gratitude for always being my best supporter.

For Gergely, Lori, Diyanna, Helen, and Belinda for your reliable and thoughtful care. I honestly don't know where I would have been without you all these past few months. I shall not forget.

Most of all though, this book is for my daughter, because however miraculous these women were, and they were, they have never once impressed me as much as she has every day through this global crisis.

Stronger, braver, wiser, and brighter than any star in the sky, my love.

Where would the world be without you, Aimée Jo?

Foreword

By Jan Kuśmirek

This book could be said to be about the bee, a people that have been with us since the dawn of time. It is about the hive, the social structure of the society of the bee people. It slips effortlessly from the bee to the relationship bees have with humankind, and the awe and respect shown to this vital insect.

This intriguing book could be said to be about the lost spiritual and cultural relationship we as humans have with the natural world, but it is more than this. Well researched and fully tempered with fact, it is far more than a didactic exercise into the world of bees, their cultural and sociological influence. Evidence of what might be termed bee culture is explored in archaeology or indeed in ancient or present comparative religion, but it's also a journey into the mystery of the divine feminine and her expression in womankind. It is about how the Queen Bee has shaped our thinking and actions, and how she still has adherents, mediators manifesting in the sterile world of today.

Elizabeth Ashley herself identifies with the Melissae, the priestesses of the cult of the sacred bee, the Queen Bee. Effortlessly we are taken to all the cult sites of importance, providing us with the accepted interpretations, but laid alongside a more physical approach, one of experience rather than an intellectual exercise.

If you want to know the legends of past civilizations or want to become more familiar with the pathways of ancient peoples, then this is certainly a book to enjoy. All the characterful goddesses are there from Inanna to Cybele, Ashtoreth to Aphrodite. Their mysteries explored not only as history but their relevance to today.

1

The hive contains both male and female and the drone is not forgotten. In Egypt, the bee becomes the tears of Ra, unusually a move away from the feminine aspect. The unifying factor of contrast, or seeming contradiction, lies in the opposites of sun and moon. The Melissae become like the bee, sometimes even reflected in their dress, often serving a variety of deities reflecting emotions, needs and desires, but with the all-important underpinning necessity for fertility. The life of a bee and the varied work they undertake in the hive is related to the varied work of a priestess.

The book carefully weaves such ideas as sacred drumming to induce trance, alongside that of the proverbial humming of bees. What is delightful too, is the sudden return from the esoteric and mythic, to the very different types of bees that exist, and the relationship or attachment they may have to the pantheon of deities. This contrast of physical to spiritual is at the heart of the writing. It is unusual to read of the everyday existence and sometimes mundane life of a priestess in the modern world of Goddess spirituality which tends to centre upon personal self-development. More narcissism, rather than change or service. True, the book ventures into the spirit realm, but equally, comes that contrast to the physical realities.

One thing that clearly emerges to the reader is the role of the Melissae as mediators between the physical world and the spirit world. Or as some would prefer between the material and spiritual world. Elizabeth Ashley leaves the reader to decide between Queen Bee and Queen of Heaven but she makes clear Melissae are still needed today to act as mediatrices between goddess and man.

Jan Kuśmirek, Founder of Fragrant Earth, Aromatherapist and Priest of Avalon

Introduction

By profession, I am an aromatherapy researcher. The Melissae of antiquity are often alluded to in ancient botanical texts about *Melissa officinalis*, the plant better known as Lemon Balm.

What had begun as an innocent desire to understand the actions of Melissa essential oil soon evolved into an obsession to understand more about these priestesses who had served the ancient Greek goddess Demeter.

Who were they? What was their function and what were they for? Their secrets have been veiled for millennia, to ensure mankind, and our planet, continues to benefit from feminine healing.

In hindsight, I feel rather silly for not recognising how powerful the magical garden was that *The Strong Silent One* (my husband, Darrell) was building around us, or for not having intuited the Bee Goddess, the most powerful Goddess human history has ever seen, was hurtling towards me faster than the speed of sound.

I didn't.

It never occurred to me for a second.

If it had, I'd likely have chucked away the innocent-looking bottle of oil that inspired my original desire to find them. Launched it, as if it were searing glass, straight from the furnace from whence it leapt.

The difficulties of telling their story are myriad, not least because this will be the first time their teachings have been written down. In some ways, since much of it is constructed in metaphor, oral tradition may have served them best. Mythical lessons land differently when you hear them than if they are read.

The main teaching of the Melissa priestesses is *bee shamanism*, delivered via Knowledge Lectures in the darkness. Heard

3

with your eyes closed, they are captured in the womb space of your mind. No-one takes notes. Everything is drawn from memory interwoven with one's own thoughts and observations. Honeyed wisdom is passed from mouth to ear, regurgitated and recapitulated.

The beauty of the work resides in its complexity. Whilst there is an architecture to it, it's as far away from "One-size-fits-all" as you can get.

Individual and quiet.

Intimate and personal.

Mystery work – as in the Mysteries of Eleusis, the domain of Demeter's Melissae priestesses – is drawn from one's own internal revelations. Peeling back layers of femininity, it reveals your part in life's mystical pattern. Through it, one recognises the sacred privilege of being chosen as Earth steward.

To become a Melissa, a woman delves deeply to find reserves of courage to experience every grain of life's pollen. Orgiastically revelling, with lusty, unbridled abandon, regardless of how bitter it may sometimes taste. Hungrily exploring its substance, she heads back to the hive to dance a mystical tale for her sisters.

Escaping to that realm has taught me to live and breathe with the greenery that resides outside my window. I have come home to myself, resting quietly amongst the flowers. Communing with the bees, I live a simpler and more beautiful existence.

According to mythology, *Meliades* were primordial nature spirits inhabiting two plants, ash trees and Lemon Balm. According to the poet, Hesiod, Meliades were the original Melissae, born from droplets of blood that fell onto Gaia, when Cronus castrated his father, Ouranus. I have three spirit guides who are Meliades.

Their names are Empedo, Melitte, and Parsnip.

Empedo might appear in one of two guises, as ascended bee priestess (she was both womb shamaness and midwife) or as freshwater nymph. Her name means steadfast. She is the serenest of the three.

Melitte is the most ancient of any consciousness I have ever worked with. She is ascended priestess, guardian of honeyed wisdom, architect of the knowledge of the district of Melitte in Athens (where the Acropolis is, in Attica, Greece), and priestess to the Cretan bee Goddess, Britomartis.

Melitte appears as one of the companions of Persephone, when she was abducted from the meadow, and as one of the Minotaur's sacrificial victims.

Parsnip is a bee spirit.

Confused? Yes, well, trust me. One thing you learn when you work with Melissa energy is when you're given a thread, sometimes it's best just to accept it. Some things have answers, others only more questions. Some things defy explanation. They just *are*.

Like bees' wings, they are veiled.

Hidden.

Outside of the weave.

Poets and storytellers famously created the Greek religion. This was the first time I had questioned how that could have come to be. Even with lessons hidden in the myths, it seems strange that poets could just turn up, tell what are essentially fairy tales, and they would be accepted as components of one of history's most influential civilizations. It's only deep study of the rituals that inspired those stories, that reveals the sheer brilliance of ancient Greece itself.

To my mind, bee shamanism seems to have reached its pinnacle around the sixth century BCE and informs vast swathes of the ritual calendar. The power of a ritual is in its weaving. A person's perspicacity comes from how they encounter it. Who they are, what their knowledge is, where their intentions are focused, and even what is happening in their life will inform the wisdom they draw from it.

The best example I can give you of that is being pregnant.

Suddenly the whole world seems to be having babies, and it's all anyone wants to talk about. Carrying a baby taps into a resonance that draws communion to you. Everyone wants to unload nightmare labour stories and to discuss their swollen ankles. Similarly, when you watch a ritual, and work with bee consciousness, awareness shifts. Suddenly bee "stuff" is everywhere. Study myths and simultaneously *search* for bee stuff and something incredible happens... you enter the world of pollination.

That's not accidental.

It's how the priestesses designed it.

Scholars believe Greek myths were written as explanations for rituals poets had seen, and the most famous of all these, did indeed, belong to the Melissae.

The Mysteries of Eleusis were highly advanced spiritual technologies. Cloaked within an extremely witty and addictive game, their primary objective seems to have been twofold: to teach how planets moved around the sky and to explore as many members of the *Insecta* class as you could.

The result was an extraordinary thirst for knowledge, a deep love for nature's mysteries, and, for those most accomplished, a release from the restrictions of space and time. Consider how small you *feel* exploring orbits and trajectories of planets, versus how enormous, witnessing aphids upon a rose.

We begin to sense the essence of Melissa teachings.

Opposite ends of a spectrum, but at some point, one merges into the other.

The enormity of the cosmos, compared to the tiniest of Earth's inhabitants.

The priestess sits between them, acting as intermediary.

Coordinated enabler of the universe. Melissa, the mediatrix.

The priestess who *feels* her way to mastery. Her edges raw, reawakened by the beatitude of all she beholds. Everything

Introduction

charmed, always fragrant and wild. Encapsulating and embodying *all* of it, recognising the healing that emerges from venomous stings.

Their stories weren't previously set down on paper because there was never a need for them to be. Our ancestors instinctively knew how to access womb wisdom. They mined peripheral information at will. Since shamanism is no longer an everyday activity, the knowledge is mostly ignored. If we are not careful, these skills will be lost for ever.

So, I wonder, will you find it easy to believe my stories?

Probably not.

I foresee being like Kassandra, the oracular priestess who betrayed Apollo's trust, whom he cursed to ensure no-one would ever believe anything she said again. I envisage sounding like a bumbling idiot. If you are open to bee thoughts, as you enter the hive though, you too might sense honey trickle in. Who knows, you might even come to appreciate this as the work of a tired, fat, and very hairy bee.

Before we get to the heavy-duty study though, I'd like to take a moment to introduce the most diligent and bossiest of my spirit guides. This book couldn't have happened without her. Ostensibly, she is its authoress. It's only fair you meet her and learn one of her funniest stories. Then, we'll begin the Melissa tale.

Her name, Parsnip, came about after a colleague said how much she was looking forward to reading this Melissa book and particularly about how the journey had affected me. I was a bit taken aback by that, because I realised that most of what I had written so far had been very evidence-based, lots of referencing, lots of proof, and it struck me, at that point, that you, the reader, couldn't really see me in the book. That was partly because I was relying solely on academic study and no intuitive stuff yet, but mainly because it has been such an intimate, strange, and rather boring-to-the-outside-world tale.

7

I had no idea how to put that right.

So, that night, before I went to sleep, I asked for guidance about how the bees thought I should move forwards. The next day was a cold, November, Sunday morning, and as I lay in bed, one of the bee priestesses paid me a visit. This one, the one who communicates with me most, is the funniest and the snarkiest, a kind of mischievous ringleader, whom I perceive as looking like a pretty cartoon stickwoman/bee in a skirt. My co-conspirator from the bee kingdom perpetually, and good-naturedly, takes the Mickey out of me. Over time I have learnt to give as good as I get.

Half awake, half asleep, as I was, she waltzed in, and interrupted me as I sorted through my dreams. As usual, she announced herself, quite without apology.

"Parsnips," she said.

"What?"

"You heard me. Parsnips."

"Well, yes. I *did* hear you, but I haven't got a clue what you're going on about. What about them?" I demanded, with irritation.

By now, you might have realised these dialogues have become rather commonplace. She and I know each other well, and our conversations flow back and forth with little recourse to manners. We relate as if we've worked together for years.

"Parsnips!" she said exasperatedly, shrugging as if it was the most obvious thing in the world.

Right.

Parsnips.

Obviously.

Got it.

Pushing her root vegetable mutterings aside, I continued to sift through my dreams of Byzantine song.

"I said… PARSNIPS!" she retorted in annoyance, tapping her tiny, ant-like foot.

"I *know* you *said* parsnips, but it makes no sense.

Why on Earth are you prattling on about parsnips?
I was enjoying lying here just thinking about music!"

"Because they're important..."

"Are they now?" said I, with resignation, already imagining the rabbit hole I'm heading down.

"Yes," she squealed, bursting to let me in on the joke, "Yes, they are..."

"Come on then. *Why* are parsnips important?"

"Because we love them," she giggled, gleefully rubbing her hands.

"You're right. I do love them. Thank you."

"Yes, we know *you* do, but *you're* not the issue. *We* really like parsnips."

"We *who*, for goodness' sake? *Bees? Bees* like parsnips?"

"Yes, of course, bees. We love them, so we make them."

"Right. OK," says I.

"I'll try and make sense of that, thank you." *Even though I haven't a clue as to why you'd choose to give me something quite so random to work with.*

I got out of bed, snuggled into my dressing gown, went downstairs, and got the laptop out.

"I just had the weirdest dream," I said to The Strong Silent One who answered with a "Hmmm?" then went back to some word game on his tablet.

On my own then, clearly.

I stared at the keyboard.

What on Earth to look up?

I googled "Bees Parsnips" because, well, what else is there?

The first few results were cake recipes and then this.

A cutting of a newspaper article entitled **"Bees Make Parsnip Seeds."**

A scientific agricultural trial showed the difference between plants artificially pollinated by people and those by bees. They proved plants grown inside a screen tent would not create seeds if pollinated by human hands. The problem, they identified, was the flowers of the umbellifer plant were simply too small. Even paintbrushes didn't quite hit the G-spot, but when left to the intentions of the bees, the vegetables generated no fewer than 15,000 seeds.[1]

Bees do indeed make parsnips!

I decided to open with this story because even my eleven-year-old son, Dexter – whose answer to anything even vaguely Melissa related is to roll his eyes and say, "You're just obsessed by bees" – even Dexter had to admit *that* was weird!

But more, it helps me to illustrate several points.

Mainly, and perhaps most importantly, everything about the bee priestesses *is* marvellously and unsettlingly strange. The magic of the Melissae priestesses is bizarre, but often mundane. That's what makes it truly miraculous. Every day bees bring something other-worldly; you simply have to notice what's happening, right in front of your face.

Incidentally, did you know that while we have just two eyes (or I guess a third eye too), bees have five eyes? The male bee, the drone, has far larger eyes than the workers. He needs them to find the queen in their nuptial flight.

Bees drink through their proboscis, taste through their feet, and smell with their antennae. They perceive everything they need to know about pollen through hairs in their abdomen. (Other species of bees also collect pollen on their hairy tummies, correctly termed their *scopa*.) Honey bees sweat wax through special glands in their lower abdomen. They mix this with tree resins collected onto their hairy bellies, then turn it into propolis to create their honeycomb structures.

And did you know bees loved parsnips?

Well, you do now.

Look how far you have come in just a few pages of the book.

Chapter 1

The Beginning of The Journey

I'd read the Melissae had been ancient Greek priestesses who had served Demeter, and perhaps other goddesses too. Listed in all herbal texts, their name appears, but nothing more.

I wanted to find them.

Who were they? What were they for? What was their association with Lemon Balm and why had they disappeared?

I'd sit in the garden, surrounded by herbs, my hands in her leaves, enjoying her company and lovely scent.

I sat for days, willing her to speak.

But she wouldn't. She'd nothing she thought I was ready to hear.

I persisted, day after day; insisted I wanted to know.

Then, one afternoon she whispered: "Change your breath."

A noise in my head. A sneaky utterance. Nothing more.

Like a glimpse out the corner of my eye.

There, but maybe not.

But no. *Definitely.* I heard her speak.

So, I did. I changed my breath.

Immediately, I knew I'd done it wrong.

I tried different breathing patterns until, oddly, I felt myself disappear.

Sliding out of this reality, I found a place that was new in my mind. A dark and intimate space.

I knew it though, because I *had* been there before; in those moments of oblivion before orgasm, and the blackness of transition before my babies were born. In that feminine space, the most sensual and arcane seemed reasonable, locked away in the darkness of the womb.

Then a train sped by, interrupted my trance, and the moment was gone. Feeling robbed and bereft, try as I might, I could not return to the space.

So, I went inside and made some tea.

The next day, scared of being outside by a dark cloud signalling rain, my calculations revealed the moon to be at her fullest in just two days.

My usual route to intuition rose in her lunar majesty on a warm, clear, and balmy night. Sitting amidst the herbs didn't feel like work at all. The hyssop, not yet flowered, smelled sensuous and bitter; the camomile, just starting to peep through. Roses and lavender held the fascination of the late evening bees, so when I stroked Lemon Balm again, no insects bothered me there.

I breathed, carefully, deeply.

Shallowly, quickly.

Counted. Nothing happened.

But as I tried, I heard a voice again. This time though, not just one, a whole chorus of chanting, to help my breathing along.

...witnessed,
We witnessed,
we witnessed,
we witnessed,
We...

The chant continued on, and as my breathing fell into line.

Long breath in, two short ones out.

Long breath in, two short ones out.

As I got the rhythm, the chant went faster, so did my breathing until I was back there, in the womb space of my mind.

So, there I was in a cave of warmth and secrecy, rapt by the rawness of the place. Enthralled by the mysterious and empty centre of my being, where everything seemed sacred and entirely possible.

I had just one question.

What the bloody hell do I do here?

I had no answers, but it seemed to me my age-old mantra may be right. If in doubt, read.

Find out what had been written.

But I'd already done that, and there was nothing. All the usual places of Victorian research had been exhausted. The medieval texts were the same. Even the ancient Greek scholars had nothing to say about the Melissae.

After months of learning about the Mysteries of Eleusis, I was still no closer to finding these women, and what in the name of all that is good and pure, did they have to do with Lemon Balm anyway?

The first clue there may be any substance to the claim that the priestesses had indeed existed, came from a chance encounter with one of the strangest and most beautiful books I've ever read. In *The Shamanic Way of the Bee*, Simon Buxton describes his initiation into bee shamanism by way of some mysterious Eastern European priestesses called Melissae.

When researching the Mysteries of Eleusis, over which Demeter's priestesses presided, I found most scholars understandably focused their attentions upon the ritual, which attracted thousands of people every year and continued to do so for over two millennia. Fixated on the secrets the ritual might contain, their studies showed zero interest in the priestesses. Some even dismissed them as mere hostesses, simply in attendance to ensure initiates were looked after, and enjoyed a good time.

But then, I discovered works of several women. I refer to their books consistently throughout my own, because their research frames the picture I can now draw, but I heartily recommend finding copies of your own if you'd like to take this work deeper, which I suspect most women will.

These are:

Portrait of a Priestess by Joan Breton Connelly. Not a cheap book – I paid £35 for a second-hand library copy – but worth every penny. Her research is astonishing, and the pictures spellbinding. The extent of Breton Connelly's exploration is breathtaking, and to my mind, deserves to be read by every woman ever born. This book became invaluable for back checking facts against stunning photographs of Grecian artefacts from around the world. Next is a smaller book, written way back in 1896 by Elisabeth Sinclair Peck. It is a much harder read, not least because modern-day reproductions of *A Study of the Greek Priestess* have text so tiny you need a magnifying glass to read it. Nevertheless, it seems like hers may have been the first work to ever focus upon understanding the role of a priestess.

So, here is our first distinction: Breton Connelly's work helps us understand who they were, Sinclair Peck explains more about their function.

Finally, Layne Redmond's book *When the Women were Drummers: A Spiritual History of Rhythm*, helps us to understand the rise and fall of the priestess. It also reminded me not to make the mistake of seeing them obscured by a 21st century patriarchal lens.

Ancient Hellenistic scholar Christiane Sourvinou-Inwood described it beautifully, when she said her own ambition was to prevent us from being "seduced by the reflections of our own minds", encouraging us to "read ancient texts through the eyes of *their* contemporary readers."

Once I removed my modern-day glasses, and replaced them with Sourvinou-Inwood's filter, things happened. First, the priestess stepped out of the shadows, The Goddess revealed herself as woman, and I began to mourn.

Mourn The Goddess, the priestess, and the woman from the past who could have been me. I grieved my disconnect from these people, so in line with the Earth and her rhythms. I regretted the detachment I felt from my cycles, and how powerless that made me feel. I lamented every woman disallowed from learning to read, for those forbidden to speak their minds, and for those generations before me who've had their lineage obscured, raped, and suppressed.

I wept for weeks. Now the grief is finally out, hopefully, I can put it into words.

We should remember that by the times of these stories, change was already well under way. They'd been whispered by campfires, sung by minstrels with lyres, for centuries, before anyone wrote them down. It's likely myths tasted much sweeter in their original forms. Female deities as sovereigns of their own realms, serving *beside* their consorts, not ministering at their behest. Even three thousand years ago, the disconnect had already begun; stories being codified into patriarchal frames. Everything in women's interior and exterior worlds would have changed, when reverence moved from the Earth to the skies.

Marija Gimbutas, one of the key authorities of the divine feminine in Eastern Europe, spoke of her reluctance to refer to societies as "matriarchal", lest that be construed as in opposition to patriarchal, and that those would have been times where Woman ruled over Man.

I agree with her stance. Those seem to have been more *egalitarian* times. Women explored their own sovereignty to become queens. Not in competition with each other, but with steely control and mastery of themselves.

That said, the part "The Patriarchy" played in robbing women of these rites of passage is in no way small. It is right and just that it should be held accountable.

Before I go further then, I feel I should make a couple of apologies.

To the men I am fortunate enough to have in my life, I would like to say I love, respect, and applaud you. However, I suspect it may be impossible for you to understand the great yearning a woman has, a gaping chasm where she knows *something* is supposed to live, but she's not entirely sure what. Or indeed what it means to be a woman living in a man's world.

Where equality means being told you should conduct your career as if you don't have children, while simultaneously parenting as if you have no job.

Where equality is, in fact, anything but.

Men rarely appear in this book. I shall not investigate the role of the Archon Basileus (a kind of mayor whose job it was to organise and participate in civic religious functions), the Hierophant, or his priests. I acknowledge their place, next to the priestess, but my interest is in the Melissae, the priestesses, and Melissa as woman.

Chapter 2

Women, Just Beeing Women.

As stated, my quest to find the Melissae began with the Lemon Balm plant, but none of the writings about the priestesses seemed to make any mention of the botanical. I finally caught a break when I discovered a work by the celebrated Greek poet Virgil. The *Georgics*, a poem revealing the secrets of successful agriculture, was his second work, from around 30 BCE.

Written in a twelve-beats-per-line rhythm known as hexameter, the *Georgics* belongs to a time where it would have been unheard of to think of planning one's horticultural endeavours without considering the movements of the stars. I was really disappointed to realise that even Virgil goes out of date, because in the two thousand years since he committed his knowledge to paper, the rising and setting times of many of the stars have shifted, due to something called the precession of the equinoxes, so they no longer relate.

Nevertheless, the *Georgics* is useful to us.

The poem is made up of a mammoth 2188 verses written in hexameter and is divided up into four separate books.

The book that interests us is the fourth, which is further separated into two parts. The first part, lines 1-280, reads exactly as you might expect an agricultural manual would, and this bit gives instructions about how best to care for your bees, and particularly, what you should do if your swarm decides to up and leave you.

But then something strange happens. The second part swaps from this sensible lecture tone into a spellbinding story; a myth. Here, we get the sense that the allegory is clearly designed to act as some sort of teaching aid. I would suggest, after almost three years working with Melissa thaumaturgy, what we start to see is the stuff he begins to pick up clairvoyantly. First you see a fact he knew, he matches it to something in historical research, then he tells us about the third piece which has been given to him, somehow in the dreamscape.

This is the Melissa three-fold path, and you can picture it a bit like a capital letter Y. You might notice it happening in my work too. It's unavoidable in this kind of work and perhaps it's a trick of the plant. What will also happen, is everything will feel right, then suddenly feel wrong, and that's because the Melissa medicine has turned. One fork in the road will take you forward, you'll come to understand this as "Apollonian", and one fork takes you backwards. You may start to understand this as Dionysian. Dionysian is the realm of Persephone, of shadows and darkness, of Freud, Jung and psychiatry, and it reads just like a myth.

Now, I've gotta tell you, reading Virgil's story feels incredibly odd, because I feel like I have gone back 40 years. It turns out this is the story of Orpheus and Eurydice, which was my absolute favourite picture book when I was a kid.

For those of you who don't know, Orpheus is this amazing lyre player who goes on these incredible adventures with Jason and his budding band of Argonauts. Potentially part of his musical brilliance derives from his parentage, since he is the son of the god, Apollo, and one of the Muses, the patron of poetry, Calliope.

As I am sure you can imagine, Orpheus is a bit of a catch. He's savvy about how to use his instrument, and according to my picture book had an impressive head of thick, black curly hair. The wood nymph, Eurydice, was not immune to his charms, and within a few weeks they had fallen head over heels in love. Soon they marry and it should all be happily ever after, but where would the fun be in that?

You see, the problem is that Eurydice's feminine wiles have also entranced the beekeeping god, Aristaeus, and he is stark staring furious that she has chosen to spend her life with someone else. "I'll teach her," he vows, and he wreaks dramatic vengeance upon her by sending a venomous snake to find and bite her.

Poor old Eurydice is wandering and, wouldn't you know it, steps upon the serpent, which does Aristaeus's bidding and sinks its fangs into her foot. Inadvertently, he has gone too far and Aristaeus realises he's killed Orpheus's beloved wife.

Well, if the beekeeping god felt pleased with the success of his vengeance, it wouldn't last very long. Eurydice's sister nymphs were furious about what he had done. Incandescent with rage, they rose from the forest, cursing him that every one of his bees should leave, and the bees, bless'em, they did exactly that. They upped and left, deserting his care.

Aristaeus is bereft. He hasn't a clue what to do, so he begs advice from his mother, the nymph, Cyrene.

She ponders for a while and then suggests her son might be best placed seeking counsel from Proteus, the prophetic old man of the sea. The passage in the *Georgics* that we're interested in is of the advice Proteus gives Aristaeus about how he might be able to assuage Eurydice's soul, and in return, how he might hopefully have some possibility of being able to recover his bees.

Proteus tells him:

So, when you look up at the swarm released from the hive,
floating towards the radiant sky through the clear summer air,
and marvel at the dark cloud drawn along by the wind,
take note: they are continually searching for sweet waters
and leafy canopies. Scatter the scents I demanded,
bruised balm *and corn parsley's humble herb, and make*
a tinkling sound, and shake Cybele's cymbals around:
they'll settle themselves on the soporific rest sites:
they'll bury themselves, as they do, in their deepest cradle.

In addition, he tells Aristaeus that he must sacrifice four cows and four bulls, which he does. After nine days, multitudes of bees spring forth and Aristaeus's hives are refilled.

Very odd.

So, here we can see the ancient Greek wisdom that [Lemon] Balm is rubbed onto hives to prevent them from flying away, and if we look at it through 21st century eyes, that is probably all we can see. However, contemporary readers would have comprehended more than we can.

First they believed that bees had a characteristic relationship with death. In particular, that they emerged from dead animals, especially cows and lions. Living in caves and arriving unheralded from small cracks in the ground, like snakes do, early people believed bees to interact with the souls of the dead, and could relay messages to and from the ancestors. Rather like Hermes, the messenger god, these liminal creatures were believed to be psychopomps moving between the worlds at will.

To the ancient Greeks, it would seem only natural that Eurydice would encounter bees in the Underworld. Of course, with the dead. Where else would they be?

The next point of interest comes in the line: *and shake Cybele's cymbals around...*

For the priestesses of Cybele were none other than the Melissae. The priestesses who led their supplicants on shamanistic journeys with the help of dancing and drums.

There she is then. We've found her. Hidden in plain sight. Our Melissa.

We should be clear...

Thanks, mainly to the Roman obsession with writing and recording, the ancient Greek priestess has been preserved, but she belonged to a long lineage of Melissae who came before and after her. At the end of their public lives, their name changed to Mellonia, priestesses of the Roman Goddess Of Honey (also known as Mellonia or Mellona), but then they seem to disappear without a trace.

However, long after, hidden away from the dangers of Rome's desire that the world should worship their Catholic God, women still gathered to worship their deities in peace.

When the Emperor Theodosius closed the sanctuaries and ordered the persecution of the Pagans in 391 CE, the Melissae buzzing quietened, guardedly, to a hum. No longer able to dance in the sunlight, our bees preferred to remain hidden in long grass and quietly, *very* quietly, whispered to The Goddess on their pollen covered knees.

Priestesses yes, but ordinary women too.

Potnia (Greek: πότνια, "mistress") is a poetic title denoting honour, used chiefly to address females, whether these be goddesses or women. The term was inherited from the Mycenaean term for goddess and encompassed a variety of female deities.

In classical Greece, the title referred to the earth Goddess Gaia (Ge), then in classical antiquity *Potnia* could apply to any one of The Goddesses: Demeter, Artemis, Athena, Hekate, and Persephone.

The epiphany or motif of Potnia is a bee.

Potentially, this may be the first time we get a feel for the vastness of the term Melissa – certainly here as Potnia, she might be a goddess, or actually one of *several* goddesses. She *could* be a priestess, but any honourable woman would qualify as *Potnia* or *Melissa*.

In places like Ephesus, reverence of the Great Mother was so strong, that after the sanctuaries closed, goddesses took on the guise of the beautiful Black Madonna, spreading across the continent, especially into France. Melissa didn't disappear; she went into witness protection and changed her name.

The line continued, especially in Eastern Europe. Modern-day Melissa teaching is called forth from English and Welsh druidic traditions and from Lithuania, where Christianity did not reach until around the 15th century, and then only in urban areas. Layers upon the surface of Paganism, especially in more rural parts of Lithuania, remain very thin; thus, the traditions that history told us had, to all intents and purposes, been lost, rather have been very privately and quietly preserved.

So why Bee?

Of all the early symbols we find, after the serpent, the most represented is the bee.

Records of "Bee Women" or "Sacred Bees" can be found much further back in time than Ancient Greece. They appear in many places throughout the prehistoric and ancient worlds, but they seem to be especially prominent in Greece, Crete, and Asia Minor.

A hurdle to overcome is if we pin the title, Melissa, to Ancient Greece, we get bogged down by their myths. We risk imagining them as primitive and childish or dismissing them as naïve. The Melissae were more than just *servants* to Demeter. Access to divine source itself, they *embodied* the Divine Feminine. As mediators of divinity, they ensured the fickle goddess of harvest remained happy.

Let's wind the clock back farther, to before civilization began. Journeying back that far, makes it easier to visualise how the Melissae might have emerged.

Palaeolithic cave paintings offer tiny glimpses of what life may have been like and give early representations of people's sacred relationship with the Earth.

Most paintings portray peaceful scenes, and whilst early man is shown wielding spears, no art from this period has been discovered where weapons are depicted as being directed at other humans. Generally, it suggests tribes lived peacefully, side by side. Survival depended on collaboration and trust, aligning with the seasons, and moving with the energies of the Earth. Communities were small only taking what they needed from the land. Mankind and nature flourished in harmony.

Perhaps unsurprisingly the most telling clues about these people are found in rock faces, given the fundamental role caves played in their lives. They offered shelter from harsh unpredictable weather but also made convenient venues to meet with neighbouring tribes. Here, intel about rich hedgerows and trees laden with food was traded in respect and care, and the congregation of our world's earliest religion gathered in the cool safety of the vagina of the Great Mother.

It was perhaps here that the association between the vagina of The Goddess and the human womb was first explored.

The womb – The dreaming vessel.

The oracular centre of the womb; the place of gnosis, of *knowing*.

Womb as a place of healing and sacred centre of divine source energy.

In *Womb Awakening*, Bertrand and Bertrand describe:

The Great Womb of Creation, the pre-existent birther of All, was once known as the Great Whore. In the Semitic languages of the Middle East, **hor** *meant "cave" or "womb." She was also known as a harlot – a "Womb of Light."*[2]

Palaeolithic shamanesses passed sacred womb cosmology from mouth to ear. They forged ecstatic rituals, blending loving appreciation for the world into a holistic system of unity.

The womb as the void of creation. The place from whence children came, birthed within the mouths of caves with sisters dancing their souls into being. To the early human mind, the cave was the external manifestation of the safest place they had ever been; the cave that had protected them as they had formed.

The womb of the tomb. The place they returned to, to wait for The Goddess to rebirth them.

The way people inter their dead portrays much about a society's perception of life and death, and the forces they understood as surrounding them.

Around 34,000 BCE, ceremonial elements began to develop in burials. Bodies were placed into foetal positions to face the rising sun in the east. Many have been found adorned with cowrie shells, an ancient symbol of the vulva.

Then around 30,000 BCE, artistic representations of vulvae seem to explode right across Europe, on cave walls, in graves, and they were often carved into amulets and jewellery. Many were carved into stone then smeared with the bloody tinge of red ochre.

Some look realistic, others more abstract; wishbone-shaped amulets with vulvic gashes carved between the legs. Some have been found in isolation, but usually, these amulets are found alongside other images of The Goddess. Rather than simply being anatomical representations, it's thought these carvings represented stories celebrating fertility, reproduction, and contemplating rebirth.

The divine being celebrated by early Man was female. Symbolism reflected her existence, her ability to autogenerate (to birth herself) and to rebirth. The vulva symbolised restoration into some new existence... perhaps some new way of being.

Archaeology suggests cave gatherings continued for thousands of years. Over time, early man began to decorate this sacred space, adorning entrances to caves with vulvae depictions. Inside they celebrated totems: bulls, snakes, birds, and bees.

Let's take a jump along the timeline. A huge one. About five millennia long...

You land somewhere special; in the sand, by your feet, is a tiny, odd-looking rock.

Look closer. Run your hands over the weathered shape and notice curves unfold beneath your hands. The rock has been carved to depict a woman.

A Venus!

Around 25,000 BCE, beautiful female figurines began to appear as far north as Siberia, right across to Italy.

The similarities between the statues are fascinating.

Humungous breasts, and gloriously wide, accommodating hips. Their dimensions are distorted, all their other features sculpted as being comparatively smaller and less significant.

When inspected closely, scholars have discovered these figurines represent many aspects of womanhood. In 1991, archaeology Professor Prudence C. Rice published that she had found that while some are depictions *of* pregnancy, others are carved with flatter breasts and narrower hips of maidens or the saggy, wrinkled breasts and buttocks of crones.[3]

Marija Gimbutas described how the vulvae of pregnant Venuses gape wide open,[4] but then Randall White, a Professor of Anthropology from New York University, described how he'd found the vaginas of these pregnant Venuses to be more nuanced than that, disclosing that what they actually seemed to depict was different degrees of dilation.[5]

So, could it be that rather than representing fertility as an abstract concept of The Goddess, these Venuses were teaching aids to educate early women about bodily changes and to demystify the arcane *process* of birth?[5]

Shawntell Nesbitt from the University of Western Ontario certainly thinks so.

Her research had been focused on French Gravettian statuettes dated to between 33,000 to 21,000 years ago. As many as 65% of the oldest Venuses depicted pregnancy, but when she compared that to Magdalenian ones, which were younger at between 17,000-12,000 years old, only about 35% depicted it.[6]

She believes this indicates early women discovered ways of *controlling* birth.

The Moon Goddess

The *Venus of Lausell*, or *Femme à la Corne* (Woman with Horn), is a bas-relief of a nude woman. She was discovered in 1911, carved into a fallen block of limestone in a rock shelter in the French Dordogne region. Standing just under half a meter tall and painted with red ochre, she is thought to have been created somewhere around 23,000 BCE and is believed to be the earliest representation of the Mother Goddess ever found.

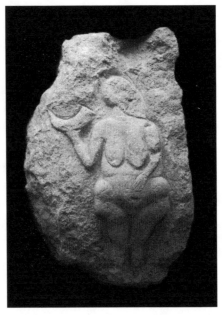

Venus de Lausall kept in the Bordeaux Museum.

She has gloriously wide hips, fleshy thighs, and a pendulous bosom. In her right hand, she holds a bison's horn: the symbol of the crescent moon.

Moon symbolism stood central to Goddess worship.

When two horns appear together, they depict the full moon cycle. Here, the shape of the cornucopia and crescent moon metaphorically align to the vulva.

Layne Redmond stated that early women, living close to the equator, menstruated in synchronicity with the moon.[7] They bled in line with lunar cycles.

In classical mythology, the **dark** of the moon (the new moon or crescent) is associated with menstruation.

The moon held three complexly interwoven ideas:

Cycles of fertility, of water, tides, and blood; the sacred fluids of most religions.

Growth and change corresponding to the phases of the moon.

Notions of birth, growth, fruition, dissolution, death, and rebirth also linked with the lunar cycle.

Hunter-gatherers marked time by watching the sky.

The sun showed hours. The moon counted days.

Watching the Heavens, they sensed the seasons, almost like the beat of a drum, and felt associations with the sun and moon.

In the darkness, time has no concept. Thoughts are fleeting, irrational, and non-linear. Where solar medicine encapsulates the world of organised thought, moon medicine embodies everything we know about feelings.

The sun radiates heat and light outwards, and the moon reflects it back. The sky's night-time Goddess stabilises our climate. She moderates Earth's wobble upon its axis. The tides are directed by her pull. Mayhap, it's her watery disposition that affects our being, drawing our moods as if waves lapping the shore. And just as she reflects daytime light, the moon is reflective of the true self, as represented by the sun.

Reflection she may be, but you could never confuse moonlight for the golden light of the sun. The moon has a different flavour, a coolness, a romantic magnetism that somehow speaks of secrets and dreams.

Strange too, how she has a propensity to surprise us, don't you think? Her solar counterpart rises and falls in predictable rhythms each day, but the moon has the power to startle, catching your eye to bear witness to the majesty of the enormous silvery orb in the sky. Because she isn't predictable, is she? She rises and sets in obscure places, riding high only on nights when we view her as full, and appearing for but a few hours when new.

The vessel through which our feelings flow, the moon governs our reflections, our responses, and reactions. Casting white light on our deepest needs, our basic habits, our instincts, and overwhelmingly, our unconscious actions too.

It's our urges, our triggers, our creativity, and inspiration. It's the difference between insular and extrovert, between spiritual or spirited, and it's the part of us no-one else can see.

To some extent, the moon carries the vibration of the sacral chakra. Where the root chakra pertains to security, feeling safe and what the child *needs*, once that has been mastered and assimilated, kundalini climbs into the sacral and speaks to the part of us that *wants*.

The moon pertains to the things in life that make us happy. Our preoccupations, our hopes, our dreams, and whimsy. On days where we just fancy something a bit different, that's the caress of the moon.

In short, the moon casts silvery light upon our shadow.

This is the walk of the Melissa, to start to understand her conscious mind, and then to draw out her shadow. In doing so, she begins to better know and understand herself, and begin her journey towards self-mastery.

This non-linear irrationality meant it was women who became the keepers of lunar knowledge, the Melissa secrets of space and time, and the shamanistic mysteries of What Is. Why *does* a woman bleed each month and not die? What miraculous power means a woman gives birth, when men are little more than bystanders in the process, except for a fateful moment that decides the difference of a pregnancy or not. What terrible nightmare decides whether the womb will bear something that lives and breathes, and indeed if it does, whether that child will make it to adulthood, or be interred to rot.

Of course, the omnipotent power of fate *must* be seen to be woman, and in terms of fertility, she *must* be pregnant.

In a cave known as **La grotte-abri de la Magdeleine des Ablis**, found in Penne du Tarn, Occitaine, France, there are extraordinary carvings of a pregnant woman, whom we assume to be the Mother Goddess, surrounded by pregnant mares and bison.

The **Mistress of the Wild Beasts** is a familiar theme appearing in many religions, especially shamanistic ones. As Mistress, the deity not only *controls* the creature but seemingly *assumes* its innate power as her own.

Captivated by animals, our ancestors passed days watching how beasts honed their species' abilities. These discoveries taught them strategic ways to improve their own.

Spiders spin intricate webs, waiting patiently until there is no way for their prey to escape. Snakes sense everything through their bellies and shed their skins to grow. Bees make hives, where the success of the organism relies on the many operating for the good of the one. Bees may be insects in their own right, but the superorganism of the colony is the creature that has the desire to swarm and reproduce. Every bee knows his or her place, working in concert to improve not only their own world, but the human world as well.

Discovering cave paintings is not easy. It requires diligence since they exist in the dark recesses of hills. Initiates plunged into deep caverns in hope of communing with tutelary spirits that may have gifts they were willing to bestow. As they extended their hands in the darkness, their fingers stretched out to reach creatures that appeared through the walls, the thin membrane between the spirit world and this one.

Some suggest early cave rituals may have originated from a desire to quieten conflicting feelings these people felt brewing inside; a kind of apology for, on one hand, adoring their animal brothers and sisters, and on the other, needing to slit their throats.

Paradox indeed, but such, as we know, is life.

Chapter 3

An Introduction to the Shamanistic Bee Symbol

It's likely people have been using shamanism for at least 100,000 years. Its origins are lost to history, but shamanistic tribes do still exist, virtually unchanged by time.

Shamanism is a methodology, rather than being a religion. A kind of ancient technology to access knowledge through different parts of our brain. Parts we all have, but most have forgotten how to use.

Fascinatingly when Inuit shamans describe their experiences to anthropologists they speak of similar experiences as shamans from Ecuador, and in turn from Guatemala or New Guinea.

The vocabulary of shamanism has been virtually obliterated in the West. So, when anthropologist, Michael Harner, began to teach and write about it, he created new terminology for people to follow. He describes how, for the most part, early people journeyed *down* to the Lower World, the realm of Mother Earth, or *up* to the Upper World, home to angels, devas, and Ascended Masters.

Harner calls the reality we exist in, Middle World, which we share with sister plants, brother animals, and grandparent rocks. In shamanism everything is seen as animate, with a life force and interdependent on sibling life forms around it. Each with equal power.

When entering non-ordinary shamanistic realities, forms are mutable and can be interchanged. Thus, the shaman is able to take on the form of Tree; indeed, to *become* Tree, and to understand how it *feels* to be Tree. He can communicate with it, whether that would be verbally or through other senses. If he senses he has lessons that could be learnt from these Other Peoples, the shaman has the capability to bring Tree, or indeed

Wolf, Bee, or any other consciousness, back to ordinary reality to take time to experience and learn from it.

Shamans move through alternate realities, by slowing brain waves, sometimes using hallucinogenic herbs, such as ayahuasca or peyote, but often this is achieved through singing, dancing, and drumming.

The Drum

The drum induces a trance state as the priestess journeys between realms. As the beat continues, it provides an earthly link to ensure she can find her way home.[7] When the regular repetitive rhythm alters, it instructs the shamaness the time to return has come.

Readers of my book, *Rose Goddess Medicine*, may remember the earliest representation of the rose was the Sumerian Goddess Inanna, who over time syncretised into Astarte, the prominent goddess of the Canaanite or Phoenician religion, her Akkadian counterpart Ishtar, Isis, and then Aphrodite and Venus as she was adopted by many different cultures.

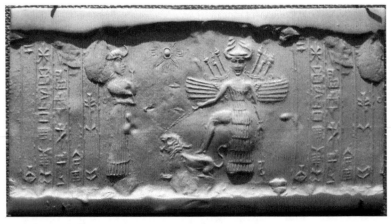

Inanna and Ninshubar. Inanna is depicted in the likeness of a bee. 2350-2150 BCE. Photograph by Sailko.

One of her legends describes how Inanna, already Queen of Heaven and Earth, decides to extend her powers even further to gain command over the underworld. She ventures down into the realm of her older sister, Ereshkigal.

Preparing for any ensuing battle, she instructs her vizier, The Goddess Ninshubur, to minister on her behalf and keep vigil for her soul. If, for any reason, Inanna does not return after three days, Ninshubur is to lament by beating her drum.

The Goddess' ritual descent takes her through seven bolted gates. Each time she reaches one, Ereshkigal demands she remove a garment, to unlock it. Finally, stripped of all her clothes, including a totem that one of Ereshkigal's nymphs found beneath the layers, Inanna stands naked before her sister and the underworld judges.

Now powerless, The Goddess is found guilty of trespassing into a realm she has no business being in. The judges offer up their sentencing. Inanna must permanently join the inhabitants of the underworld; she too must die.

Slaughtered, her rotting carcass is left hanging, swinging upon a meat hook to decay.

On the third day, Ninshubur begins her lament.

Wailing, she beats her drum.

Hearing Ninshubur's lament, the water god Enki decides he should intervene and rescue Inanna. He sends two sexless spirits down to the underworld in a bid to secure her return.

The Goddess is carried back to land by flood tides. Furious demons chase in her wake. Having delighted upon the soul they have devoured, they are determined not to relinquish it. Murderously, they chase her, resolute that if she *is* to escape, they will not be short-changed. Someone else's soul must take her place.

Meanwhile, back on Earth, it hasn't taken Inanna's consort, Dumuzid (Tammuz), long to show his colours. Seeing her absence as his chance, he exploits the power vacuum and usurps her throne. Predictably, Inanna is none too pleased, and by return, seizes her opportunity, cursing him to replace her in the underworld. Luckily for him, his loyal sister, Gestinanna, bargains to take his place, which she then does for six months out of every year.

The story of Inanna's descent dates to around 2100 BCE. Ninshubur's drumming speaks to the incredibly ancient shamanistic ideal of bringing spirits back from the underworld or guiding them back to the place of the living. Today, the assistant still drums whilst the shaman is in trance. As the journey closes, and the drumbeat changes, the shaman is reminded it is time to return to the land of their birth.

Later, we'll see how this myth also expresses symbolism comparable to several other myths including that of Demeter and Persephone. However, Gestinanna and Ninshubur express the earliest ideals of the Melissa priestess, she who understands the power of the rhythm of the drum, and she who would self-sacrifice to interact with the underworld, for the good of others.

The Grain Mother

Musician Layne Redmond's specialist area of historical research was frame drums as depicted signs of the ancient Goddess. Her search for the original priestess drum took her to modern-day Asian Turkey. There, she found cave paintings of the Great Goddess imbued with the qualities of prehistoric animals, insects, and birds.

This area hosted one of the earliest known civilizations.

Around 10,000-8,000 BCE, the ice age glaciers melted. Water levels rose to around 300ft above sea level. Animals were swallowed by the soggy ground. The great thaw threatened human existence. With their primary food source of meat gone, people headed up into the mountains and began to supplement their diet with grains. Philosopher Irwin Thompson described that "women and children could collect in three weeks, enough grain to feed the family for a year."

Naturally, challenges accompanied this boon. A means to store it was required, but if you set up a barn, you also need to remain close by. This agricultural development marks the beginning of farming and the first permanent communities. Mythology expert, Joseph Campbell, described how the environment the shaman found himself in influenced how his gods developed. When hunters worked in isolation, their deities and spirits had more nebulous and whimsical natures. Agrarian societies developed religions that were far more complex.

Archaeologists have uncovered two important early cities that flourished for many thousands of years in Asia Minor (the area we now refer to as Turkey), Çatalhöyük and Hacilar.

The height of Çatalhöyük's power was around 7000 BCE. It doesn't seem to have had any municipal buildings, only domicile residences clustered tightly together. Analysis of skeletal remains shows three distinct racial types coexisting together. They raised cattle and sheep, made earthenware vessels for cooking, eating, sprouting grains, and holding mead. It paints a picture of people living in close-knit communities; helping each other, trading together and even marrying within these groups.

As is often the case, death most articulately betrays the stories of the living. The inhabitants of Çatalhöyük practised excarnation. Bodies were left out in the sun for vultures to pick dry. Clean skeletons were ritually buried in pits beneath floors and especially under hearths. Decapitated bodies were tightly bundled into reed baskets. Men's bodies were found interred with their tools, and archaeologists would come to recognise a woman's body by her accompanying spindles.

It may be that heads formed parts of separate rituals since several have been found buried at other sites away from the main complex.

Dutch archaeologist, James Mellaart, spent four seasons excavating Çatalhöyük in the 1960s. His work revealed a community religion, created by priestesses worshipping a Mother Goddess. It is believed to have thrived for over 2000 years.

The hierarchy of the household was implicit: mother, daughter, father, son. Women's sleeping quarters were raised above men's and turned to face east. Several women's bodies were found painted in red ochre, as well as that of just one man.

Each house excavated had a grain bin, displaying their staple food. Grain planting likely followed moon cycles. Seeds germinated in earthenware pots, formed in images of The Goddess. Doubtless, sacred breadmaking secrets were passed by women to their daughters.

Fertility symbolism expanded.

The water and blood of life, the nurturing milk of the breast, now also encompassed the nourishing goodness of grain. The bread oven came to represent the Great Mother's womb, and bread was transmuted into The Goddess' body.

Many later great religions featured baking bread as holy. In Sumer, temple complexes housed kitchens, set aside solely for the production of sacred loaves. Excavations of other cultural sites in Mesopotamia have uncovered ceramic bread moulds of The Goddess offering her breasts.

Women collected grain. Wheat was sorted from the chaff using a winnowing sieve. It is believed that from this, the frame drum and tambourine developed.

One of the oldest Sumerian words for drum, also means grain sieve. In Egypt, the hieroglyph which means both "cycle of time" and "drum", also shares a third meaning – "grain".

Several glorious murals were uncovered at Çatalhöyük. One, in the shrine room, depicts two groups of people dressed in leopard skins, all playing percussion. One group dances around a stag, and the second around an enormous bull. A figure holds a bull horn in one hand, and a frame drum in the other.

Again, although Çatalhöyük's murals show animals being captured, there are no depictions of killing. Perhaps the most poignant is of a powerful, pregnant Goddess, arms raised, legs spread, giving birth. She seems linked with the four classic shamanistic animal powers: the vulture, the bull, the leopard (or lion), and the bee.

Myths and community rituals developed, as a means of guiding, training, and initiating the shamans into happier and more successful lives. Women with natural abilities of accessing non-ordinary realities, both through their intuition and dreaming, became instructresses in how to journey from one reality to another.

The embodiments of natural cyclical order, women's bleeding echoed the moon. By day, the sun's journey across the sky communicated what they should be doing in the fields and in the wider world at large. As they felt the sun grow hotter on their faces, and the soil warm under their feet, they listened to the sounds of the breeze. Some days it roared through the trees, others it seemed to whisper. On days when bees emerged from their hives, it informed relative temperatures and became their barometer. They noticed that on certain days the world had specific energies, and somehow, they began to predict what days and at what moments things might happen. Perhaps, in a way, this was why rituals became so important. When life has a ritual template, it stops days from slipping. It keeps count.

Each day, the same ritual, and each moment they noticed how the world changed and what things happened around them. What flowers came out, when they died, when certain insects emerged and which predators that, in turn, coaxed out.

They observed great surges of energy as trees ejaculated seeds into the atmosphere and noticed that lions became seemingly oblivious if they snuck up as they copulated on the plains. Over time, a predictable energy became obvious as surging through all of life. A dynamic but foreseen rhythm where, one by one, each creature embraced their orgasmic life force seemingly structured by the sun.

Over time, they would come to understand that, just like their own kind, there were sexual differences between things. Sometimes two sexes, in the case of the bee, they thought three. They began to sense a pattern, which would later inform every aspect of their religion.

Melissa...

It wasn't till as late as the 19th century, that scientists were able to make sense of how properties of flower pollen and bee enzymes combined to eventually make honey. It's not hard to imagine how honey mysteries created symbolism with such a rich and potent past.

Foremost in ritual symbolism, bees represent life, birth, death, and reincarnation. Since colonies are ruled by queen bees, it would perhaps seem predictable they would align with the sacred feminine. Paradoxically though, it seems the ancients believed hives were run by *King* Bees.

Collecting nectar from flowers and turning it into golden nourishment, bees became symbols of divine wisdom. Similarly, the priestess collects wisdom from life's diversity and from it extracts her spiritual gold.

One Çatalhöyük mural depicts sumptuous honeycombs, replete with chrysalises in various stages of egg, nymph, bee and then hatching as a butterfly. Many images at Hacilar depict The Goddess wearing a beehive on her head. The tiara dubs her Queen Bee and suggests she oozes the sweetness of honey.

In Malta, The Hypogeum of Hal Saflieni was built in around 3000 BCE. A subterranean sanctuary and necropolis, it contained the bones of some 7000 bodies, when it was discovered in 1902. The temple structure utilises careful light projections from the surface level, penetrating the lower chambers. At midwinter, light streams into one of the main chambers known as the Holy of Holies. It is thought that, originally, the temple began as a cave and, using flints, obsidian, and antlers, little by little the people chiselled deeper and deeper into the soft limestone. Constructed over three levels, it looks as if developments of the temple gouged further down into the rock over time.

Items recovered from the site include carved figures of humans and animals, intricately decorated pottery vessels, amulets, beads, shell buttons and axe-heads.

Enigmatic patterns have been daubed using red ochre onto the ceiling. Amongst the spots and spirals are wonderful stretches of honeycomb. Depictions of human figures range from abstract to realistic. They seem to venerate the dead and describe the transformation of humans' spiritual existence. Notably, one strange pottery bowl shows on one side cows, pigs and goats, and the other hatched animals hidden within sophisticated geometric patterns.

Most beautiful of the finds is the Sleeping Lady, a clay figure thought to be the Mother Goddess; voluptuously fleshy, she lies on her side, apparently tranquilly dreaming.

The middle chamber of the Hypogeum, known as the Oracle Room, exhibits the most extraordinary acoustics. In his book, *Malta and its Recently Discovered Prehistoric Temples*, William Arthur Griffiths says that when something is announced within the Oracle Room, the sound is:

> magnified a hundredfold and is audible throughout the entire structure. The effect on a building full of disciples must have been electrifying, as the Oracle's words thundered back and forth through the dark.

The walls of the room, which is also thought to have been used for chanting and praise, resonate sound at a frequency of 110 Hz, a wavelength speed well known for creating an out of body experience. Oddly, 110 Hz is also the frequency of buzzing a colony of bees makes in its celebration that it is about to swarm.[8]

Malta clearly came to have a special significance to the ancient Greeks, who would come to lovingly refer to it as *Melita*, The Honeyed One.

That bees lived in caves seems to have mesmerised ancient people. Like snakes, bees have venom, and they appear from holes in the ground at predictable times of the year. However, the motifs of bee and snake say different things. Today, snake might oftentimes be seen as having malevolent intent; bees, however, have always been associated with beneficence.

Emerging from gloomy recesses, it was concluded bees must be new souls heading to the earth plane to be reborn. Sophocles seemed to know this when he wrote: "The swarm of the dead hums."

I love to imagine these early priestesses, doing what so many beekeepers have done for thousands of years since, peering into their hives. Warm, still days, scented with the fragrance of blossom, birds singing in the trees; mellow moments thinking about the bees. For the ancient Greeks though, it wasn't just the bees, or even their honey either, the honeycomb itself intrigued them. Followers of Pythagoras meditated on how the strange hexagonal phenomenon is so immaculately created with such efficient use of geometric space.

As blackbirds chased their mates around the field, perhaps these early peoples noted that the bull wasn't the only sexual champion, but also how few drones were needed to fertilise the thousands of eggs the queen bee lays each day. (Or as Aristotle once mused, trying to suss bee sexuality, maybe it was the workers who performed that deed?)

Today, we understand that a hive will overwinter with around 10,000 bees, all of whom are female. Then when the first spring flowers open to reveal their pollen, and bees start taking it back to the hive, the queen is triggered to begin laying again. This is a poignant moment both organically and mythologically, because in a colony where there were no drones, the queen generates the first males for the hive. The size of the colony will increase through the summer, from that initial 10,000, to around 60,000 bees. Only several hundred of those will be drones, whose sole proven role is to inseminate the year's new emerging queen, their sister.

The queen and drone consummate their union, surging towards the brightness of the sun, and mating in the blissful solar heat. The mating frenzy results in the drone bee's death. As he withdraws, the lower part of his body gets ripped away and is left inside the queen. Spent, his life purpose complete, the drone dies, having sacrificed himself for the good of the colony. Hot on his tail, the next drone rips out his predecessor's member, takes his turn to mate, then also plummets to his death.

I'm sure many generations of men have enviously wondered how male bees got so lucky, to have such pampered lives with nothing else to do but eat honey and have sex!

The drone function fulfilled, the remainder are allowed to stay until the end of summer, the workers seem to love having them around. Perhaps it's their lovely sonorous bass hum that pleases them? Nevertheless, in the later summer, the girls kick them out, reducing the number of bees who have to try and get through winter back to around 10,000 again. Summer worker bees have a life cycle of around six to seven weeks. Winter bees will live around six months, ageing far slower with less foraging to do. A healthy queen can live for between three to five years.

When birds huddle in nests and newts dive down to the pond floor, bees head inside to shelter from the cold. Relentlessly fanning their wings, their winter work is to maintain a hive temperature of 95 degrees Fahrenheit, so it can continue to produce honey. Throughout the winter they will graze on their gathered sweetness, only rarely venturing outside to pop to the toilet! (Bees are immaculate creatures and wouldn't dream of soiling their hive.)

As the biting frost passes, bees gingerly test the temperature outside. When the sun can generate ambient heat of around 14 degrees Celsius (58 degrees Fahrenheit), they head outside to gorge themselves on early crocuses, snowdrops, hellebores, and pussy willow catkins. That first pollen re-triggers the cycle, instructing the queen to start laying again.

Utilising sperm she conserved in her internal sperm bank – her *spermatheca* – she begins work on regenerating the hive. Using her feet as callipers, she measures the width of each comb cell as a means of deciding which egg to lay. A larger cell means more room for a drone to grow, so she drops in an unfertilised egg. Smaller cells are better for worker bees, so this time she opts for the sperm to reach the egg, fertilises it and drops it into the cell to grow.

Eggs hatch into larvae after three days. The kind of bee the queen decided the egg will be, dictates the length of time it will take the nymph to mature. The larvae that the workers have fed up to become queens are fully-grown within 16 days; drones develop in under 24 days, and it will take female workers 21 days to develop from larva to pupa.

Over the period of her lifetime, a worker bee carries out every job in the hive, instructed by pheromones and a simple understanding of life's natural order and how it should be. Understanding the efficiency of the hive will also inform our understanding of the priestess later.

Based on the number of days after hatching, these roles are:

Days 3-16 ... Mortuary Bees

The first few days of a newly hatched bee's life are spent removing the colony dead. It's profoundly moving to behold. The mortuary bee securely holds the deceased by one of its "hands", soars up and out of the hive, carrying it like a tiny angel on the wing. They progress skyward, rising up out of their frames, then descend gently, placing the corpse upon the surface of our pond. Sometimes, I wonder if they know when the lid's going to open, because it's so opportune I see it happen.

I don't have words enough to say how beautiful it is. It makes my heart ache to witness it.

I'd been told to expect several dead bees in front of the hive, but I've only found one so far. For some reason, my bees always get placed very reverently into watery graves.

There is a saying that you should always bury bees, but I rarely get the chance since there always seem to be tongues waiting greedily below. Dead bees hastily get snaffled for dinner by the newts.

It seems incomprehensible to me that even without our advanced scientific instrumentation the ancients may have understood that it was the youngest bees that performed the role, since they associated both old souls and new with psychopomp bees suggests, to me at least, that maybe they had.

Days 4-12 ... Drone Feeding

Drones are incapable of feeding themselves, until they are about four days old, after which time they just head up to the honey and simply help themselves. Until then, they are fed by nurse bees.

Days 7-12 ... Queen Attendants

These bees have the great honour of grooming the queen to spread her fragrance around to reassure the other bees that the queen is healthy and in attendance. This is called Queen Mandibular Pheromone or QMP. Whilst the name suggests it is solely secreted from her mandibles, recent research shows she also employs other body parts to secrete "backup" pheromones should that one fail.

Days 12-18 ... Pollen Packing

When foragers return with pollen, it needs to be stored in a cell. It is placed into honeycomb then mixed with a little honey to prevent it from spoiling. This *"bee bread"* will eventually be used to feed the brood.

Days 12-35 ... Honey Sealing

The bees take honey, dry it to the correct water content, and then cap it. To do this, worker bees secrete wax from glands in their abdomen and then manipulate it into sheets.

Days 12-35 ... Honeycomb Building

Honeycomb builders receive wax from other bees and use it to start building yet more comb so that the colony will be able to expand.

Days 12-18 ... Water Carriers and Fanning Bees

Water bees carry liquid from nearby pools and fluid sources to spread onto the backs of fanning bees, who in turn use their wings to fan evaporated water around the hive to keep it cool. Together these effectively operate as an internal air conditioning system.

Days 18-21 ... Guard Bees

Guard bees hover at the entrance of the hive, protecting it from unwanted visitors such as hornets, wasps, or robbing bees from other hives. How many guard bees stand sentry varies depending upon the season and how much traffic is coming in and out at any time.

Days 22-42 ... Foraging Bees

The final days of their life will be spent outside of the hive in blissful communion with the fragrance of plants. Travelling within a five-mile radius, foragers collect pollen, nectar and propolis for the hive.

Perhaps the priestess abilities are best understood by the highly evolved extra senses that bees have. We know about their five eyes, but did you know they don't have ears? No need, they sense sound through the entirety of their bodies, especially through their antennae and through the delicate hairs all over them. Their skills defy the usual parameters of time and space. Their circadian clocks are so exquisitely developed, they are capable of getting a precise fix on any bloom percolating nectar, right across their foraging radius.

So, the forager lustily plunges her proboscis deep into the orifice of flowers, feasting on fragrant juices. Sucking, licking, and frolicking in the sensual majesty of the bloom, she kneads it with her feet, quickly becoming smothered in powdery gold.

When she finds a good source of pollen, she returns to tell the rest of the hive, in order to recruit more helpers to the harvest. Dancing back and forth, she communicates, ecstatically vibrating, as she dances round in a figure of eight shape, that produces a "sound" of 250 oscillations per second (250 Hz). It's actually the movement of their wings that creates the sound we hear as their "buzz". The waggle dance also indicates approximately what angle from the hive the food source can be found, and how far away. It's believed they might even communicate how many bees they think it will take to harvest the plant.

Pollen is the most extraordinary substance. It is a complete food containing 40% protein and the entire DNA line of the blossom from whence it came.

They work together until the entire species has been pollinated, then they'll move onto the next. They can carry almost their own weight in pollen, that they smooth into tiny baskets on the back of their legs called corbiculae.

Each beehive has a solid "dance floor" close to the entrance, made up of empty cells that vibrate when a bee begins to dance. This vibration, that can be heard in every corner of the comb, is a faultless means of communication. Without it, the other bees would probably miss these vital foraging messages.

Remind you of anything? It kind of reminds me of Malta's Hypogeum, but that would be too weird, right?

Oh, reader, you ain't seen nothing yet.

It's a sad but beautiful thing that a bee will never taste the honey of her own efforts. That will come to fruition long after her 40-something days lifetime. That everything a bee does is for the good of the community, is a common theme in many religions. Saint John Chrysostom perhaps said it most beautifully, in 400 CE, when he wrote in his twelfth homily, *"the bee is more honoured than other animals, not because she labours, but because she labours for others."*

We've absorbed an awful lot of information in those few pages, so let's just find a beautiful flower, rest for a while, and ponder a little more on the nature of Bee. For the more you bear witness to the intricacies of the insect's nature, the better you understand the nuances of the Melissa priestess and her cult.

Currently, there total around 16,000 species of bee, all descended from one common lineage. They belong to the genus Hymenoptera which contains the other species of sawflies, wasps, and ants. In sum, this encompasses about 150,000 living species and 2000 more that are sadly now extinct. These 16,000 bee species can be divided into seven biological families. Some, like honey bees, bumblebees, and stingless bees, are social, living in colonies. Carpenter bees, leaf-cutter bees, sweat bees and mason bees are all solitary creatures. It is these lovelies that we create bee hotels out of bamboo canes and pinecones for.

Common features of the Hymenoptera species include the special ovipositor, the anatomical part females use to insert eggs into their mates. In bees, this ovipositor has evolved to be modified into a stinger. Young Hymenoptera creatures develop through *holometabolism*, which means that they experience a complete metamorphosis within their lifetime. Beginning as a worm-like larvae, evolving into inactive pupae, then fully maturing into bees.

As a genus they have a raft of methods of sensory and cognitive communications. Bumblebees, for example, can discern different colours and honey bees are capable of perceiving ultraviolet. If you are thinking of the bees when choosing plants for the garden, know they like pink, blue and yellow flowers the best.

Scent, of course, is extremely important to them, and indeed even within the hive there is an extremely complex pheromone signalling system.

As previously stated, bees communicate by dancing. The waggle dance she uses to recruit more bees resembles the figure of eight infinity sign, the lemniscate. It's thought the bee communicates how much nectar is procurable by how long she dances. The angle she performs it, broadcasts to her colleagues which way to fly. Scientists now wonder if there could be even more to her dance. That when she dances, perhaps some kind of odour plume might be secreted from her abdomen, portraying yet deeper information about the bountiful plant it came from.

The entire mechanism seems to depend on fragrance. Studies using simple sugar water show that if there isn't a scent, the system falls apart, and the bees struggle to identify their designated flowers. The same applies to cloudy days; bees rely upon the sun to navigate successfully. Their entire occupation depends on the weather.

They best enjoy warm, still, sunny days: if the wind's too strong, if it's raining or too cold, bees prefer to stay in their hives and wait for weather more clement.

But the bee, they say, can predict what weather is coming.

An old rhyme reads:

When bees to distance
wing their flight

The days are warm and
skies are bright
But when their flight
ends near their home
Stormy weather is sure to
come.

Thunderstorms stir up trouble. If they sense they are imminent, bees become agitated and aggressive, perhaps sensing electrical changes in the air before the storm. Bees' moods are "positively" related to temperature, barometric pressure, solar radiation, and humidity, and are "negatively" related to wind speed. Challenging weather makes them aggressive. Allegedly, bees are at their most aggressive if it's hot and humid or if there is too little wind.

Light winds are best for gathering nectar and bees normally cruise at speeds of around 15 to 20mph. Any stronger than this makes their job that much harder, because, whilst a foraging bee can tackle a strong headwind by simply flying harder, this burns most of the sugars she's consumed, wasting them. She'll have far less to contribute to the honey flow.

Rain's a pain too, because our ladies can drown in heavy downfalls, but more importantly it washes nectar off flowers. It's so diluted that by the time the bees reach it, it's barely any use at all. A forager needs to make so many journeys back and forth from the hive that to all intents and purposes she's operating at a loss.

Likewise, nectar needs to be relatively warm and loose. The colder it is, the more solid and difficult it can be to get at. Most bees seem to disappear from the garden when the weather drops to around 14 degrees Celsius. Work seems most appealing at temperatures above 16 or 17 degrees (around 60 degrees Fahrenheit).

Bee Pheromones

The industry of the hive is entirely communicated and run by pheromones. It's a fascinating topic that could take up a whole book on its own, so I'll zone in on just a couple of the most relevant to us.

The queen secretes *Queen Mandibular Pheromone (QMP)* as she walks across the comb, which is then picked up by the worker bees who spread it around the hive. As long as the hive can smell QMP, they're reassured of the health of the queen. Knowing that, they recognise that the hive is **"Queen Right"**, so there's no need to cultivate new queen cells or swarm. As she ages, the queen makes less of the pheromone, triggering, of course, the necessity to begin feeding up new larvae to become queens.

Worker bees secrete *footprint pheromone*, from their feet, so their sisters can tell which flowers they have already been to. This, in turn, enhances the *Nasonov* pheromone as they search for nectar.

Nasonov is probably the best known honey bee pheromone and is exclusive to worker bees. To free it, the bee elevates her abdomen, flexes its tip downwards then wafts it about by fanning her wings.

It has many functions in their communications, but its main property is that it's irresistibly attractive... bees absolutely delight in its fragrance.

Worker bees fan its fragrance all over the hive entrance, to welcome home foragers. Likewise, when new ones set off on their maiden training flights, older bees disperse it into the air, to teach the newbies how to come back to the hive and to guarantee everyone else returns happily with sweet bounty.

Nasonov is also used to mark the best plants to forage. Recent studies suggest it may also form part of the decision process that worker bees use to select and mark larval cells to rear as new queens. Seemingly, they discharge Nasonov onto certain cells to denote which they think should be gorged with royal jelly.

Nasonov is also used to direct swarms to their new home.

Swarms are enigmatic, fascinating, and beautiful things. A colony swarms when it feels it has a new queen ready to hatch that will be strong enough to support a second colony. Thus, the old queen and half the bees move out to find a new home. Before they leave though, they gorge themselves on honey and so, if you ever encounter a swarm, they are actually very safe things. It's as if they have just feasted on Christmas day and are way too full and blissed to be the slightest bit bothered about hurting anyone.

As they leave the hive, scout bees head off to find a new source and they land near a good hole in a tree or box. They return back to the others, do a waggle dance to tell them where to go, then return to the spot to secrete Nasonov. The bees then follow their favourite fragrance right up to their new home.

Nasonov secretion composes seven volatile compounds:

(E)-citral, (Z)-citral, geraniol, nerolic acid, geranic acid, (E-E)-farnesol, and nerol.[9]

The main constituents of Melissa essential oil are: citral (geranial and neral), citronellal and geraniol.

Almost identical.

So, it seems that Virgil may have known what he was talking about when he said that if you rub the inside of a hive with Melissa, it should stop the swarm from leaving, and indeed empty hives are baited for swarms using Lemon Balm or the cheaper lemon grass that has a similar citral dominant chemical profile. It smells like Nasonov that tells them, "Follow me. This is home. You are loved and welcome."

If a swarm happens to land on your property, ancient wisdom says you should tang them into the hive. That means tap on something that sounds like an empty log, which also speaks to percussion instruments that Virgil also described being played for a very early bee goddess, Cybele.

If it's an empty space – log or hive – that smells of Melissa, it's home.

Traditional knowledge says bees go calm if you put Lemon Balm stalks in your smoker. I'd concur with that, but then I also put lavender stalks and myrrh in my smoking mix so there are lots of sedative volatiles in that concoction anyway. Ancient wisdom says bees aren't likely to sting you if you've rubbed Lemon Balm leaves on you. I got a bee stuck in my hair, but she wasn't at all placated by me rubbing Melissa on my head in the hope that she wouldn't sting me. She gave me a right old whacker on the top of my head. I was expecting it to hurt for days (I couldn't move my eyebrows without it killing me, so everyone kept trying to make me laugh!), but I followed the herbal advice to spit on the leaves and rub them on, and the pain had gone by morning, which is much faster than expected, and my goodness, I slept well! I didn't have Melissa on me either time I got stung, nor had I smoked the bees, but I certainly wouldn't say that was proof of Lemon Balm's efficacy.

All the way through this research, I have had the sense that the Melissae must have smelt of the plant, but I can find no evidence that they did. Over time, I have come to suspect this may have been one of the key secrets of Eleusis. We'll talk about it a bit more when we look at the attire of a priestess and her cosmetics later, but I will warn you, I think the priestesses deliberately hid the Lemon Balm secret for good. What are remarkable though, as you will discover as the book unfolds, are clear parallels between what the bee pheromones do and what the Melissa duties were.

Finally, for this section, even though there are bookcases of bee facts I could add, there is an old English tradition of "Telling the bees": that any titbits of news about the family, or nuggets of wisdom should be told to the bees. Births, deaths, and marriages should all be whispered to the hive. One lady told me how she remembered her uncle had been arrested on some drunken charge, and she was flabbergasted at her grandmother's response: "Whatever shall I tell the bees?" The hive should be taken to marriage ceremonies, and if that's not possible, then you should always leave them a slice of wedding cake.

Tradition dictates that when a beekeeper dies, the bees *must* be told, the hive should be wrapped in black crêpe, and then turned to face east. Many tales tell of how the sound of the hive alters when the bees receive the awful news of their keeper's death, changing to a low, sorrowful hum. One story I heard tells of the bees actually following the hearse all the way to the church, then waiting outside during the service. Others tell of households where nobody concerned themselves with the news about someone dying (or weddings and divorces), and the decline this oversight had brought. When another family member realised what might be going on and stepped in to redress the issue by breaking the news, stories tell how the colony came back into balance.

Chapter 4

The Bee Goddess

Palaeontology pays testimony to mud swallowing millions of animals as the ice age thawed. Meat was likely very scarce. Grain was cultivated to supplement it. This rich bounty, and that the harvest could be stored and preserved, was seen as a primal grace for early Eurasian societies. In Babylonia, the goddess Ishtar was celebrated as "Lady of the Grain Store" and illustrated as a bee. Later, the Greeks would tell how Demeter taught the people of Eleusis how to cultivate grain, in gratitude for their care for her while she mourned the loss of her daughter. The myth would be acted out in ritual at the Eleusinian Mysteries.

Of course, permanent habitation brought its own problems: envy, competition, and jealousy. Eventually, peacetime would be shattered by war. Societies were crushed as armies invaded and destroyed entire districts. Men were taken prisoner, women raped, children molested, and worship of patriarchal sky gods was forced upon ever spreading regions.

Subversion transformed the Anatolian Goddess of Çatalhöyük as she merged with other cultures. Right across the Aegean, orgiastic dancing, prophesying, and drumming accompanied worship of the Mother Goddess.

Eventually in Phrygia (modern Turkey) she emerged as The Goddess Cybele (Kebele – meaning "from a cave"). Mistress of the Wild Nature, a fertility Goddess and protectress in times of war, Cybele's origins are incredibly ancient. She is perhaps the only Goddess ever worshipped there and her beginnings probably date back to the Hittites.

Images of Cybele in the second millennium BCE show her surrounded by drumming women. Layne Redmond explains,

"Priestesses of historical descendants of this ancient bee Goddess – Demeter, Rhea, Cybele – were called Melissae, that ancient word for bees." At this point in history, the bee Goddess is seen as the giver of honey, but during these violent times, her capacity for using venom underpinned her protective and retaliatory prowess.

Cybele's origin story is incredibly strange. Phrygian myth describes how some of Zeus' sperm leaked onto the Earth as he slept, impregnating Gaia. Cybele was born from the union, in the form of a hermaphrodite, Agdistis, whose multigendered being embodied all of creation. Threatened by the sheer power of Agdistis' androgyny, Dionysos was persuaded to kill them. After giving them a sleeping draft, he tied Agdistis' foot to their penis as they slumbered. Horrifyingly, when they awoke and stood, poor Agdistis ripped their member from their body. Blood poured from the injury and where it touched the soil, an almond tree sprouted from the ground.

One day, a girl, the daughter of Sangarius, the river god, was gathering fruits in the trees. She found an almond (or some accounts say pomegranate) and clutched it to her breast, and she in turn became impregnated with Attis, the Phrygian God of Vegetation.

Attis grew into the most beautiful man who utterly bedazzled poor Agdistis who was transfixed. Alas, his family had ambitious plans that he should marry the daughter of the king of Pessinus. Dutifully, he consents to do so.

But as the day arrived and the wedding march commenced, Agdistis dramatically appeared before them. Every wedding guest was driven insane by their overpowering presence, including the king and Attis, who both castrated themselves and the poor bride who sliced off her own breasts.

Full of remorse, Agdistis repents and begs Zeus to promise that Attis' body will always be preserved and never decompose or disappear. Later, in his travel guides, Pausanias would relate that Attis' body was supposedly still interred in Mount Agdistis, in Pessinus, Phrygia.

Attis was celebrated as having been born on December 25th at the winter solstice, was said to have been crucified and risen again on March 25th. Later, the Church agreed the festival of Christ's resurrection should be celebrated at the same time. The coming of spring. Some authorities suggest the castration means that Cybele is created from Agdistis. Others view Agdistis and Cybele to be separate, yet others see them as the same. Regardless, we should notice a correlation here, spring comes and so does the bee Goddess. We will see this repeatedly in myth.

The priests of Cybele, *the galli*, were eunuchs. The Celtic Gauls settled in Galatia when they conquered central Anatolia in around 277 BCE, but this name for the priests is probably far older than that. It could be that the word *Galli* relates to the word the Greeks used for Gaul and was then retained by Latin writers.

There is more written evidence of the practices of Galli than the Melissae, but references are still sparce. Most are Roman, dating to around the end of the second and beginning of the third century CE, so certain aspects of their history might plausibly have been exaggerated.

In 1977, a Dutch religious historian, Professor Maarten Vermaseren, made a summary of the scant evidence remaining about these transgender priests, in his book, *Corpus Cultus Cybelae Attidisque*. In this passage he describes what happened when a Galli priest initiated himself on The Roman Day of Blood, celebrated on March 24th.

It reads:

On the Day of Blood (dies sanguinis) he forever discarded his male attire; henceforth he wore a long garment (stola), mostly yellow or many-coloured, with long sleeves and a belt. On their heads these priests wore a mitra, a sort of turban, or tiara, the cap with long ear-flaps which could be tied under the chin. ... They also wore their hair long, which earned for them the epithet of "long-haired"; they sometimes dedicated a lock of hair to The Goddess. By preference they had their hair bleached. ... On the day of mourning for Attis they ran around wildly with dishevelled hair, but otherwise they had their hair dressed and waved like women. Sometimes they were heavily made up, their faces resembling white-washed walls.

The festivities of The Goddess were orgiastic. Their music was loud with drums and tambourines. Marauding through the streets, they screamed their utterances of praise and danced corybantic rites. They filled the streets with the sounds of the drum and cymbal, said to be imitations of Cybele's voice, as the buzzing of the bee itself.

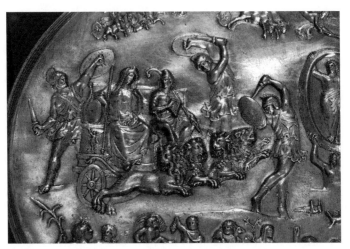

Cybele and Attis surrounded by Corybants. Milan Museum. Photograph by Giovanni Dall'Orto.

Each year on 24th March, new priests would be initiated, as they, too, tore off their own genitalia. It is unclear whether castration was limited to the penis or included their testicular sacs, but it seems likely to me at least, that the drone's sacrifice for loving his queen was enacted, so that he too could become one of her sterile servants.

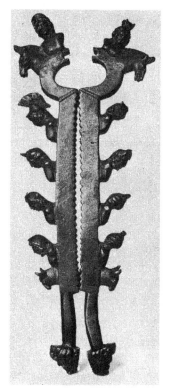

Believed to be a castration clamp for the Cult of Cybele. It is decorated with figures of Cybele and Attis, while the days of the week are represented by busts of other Roman deities. Found in the River Thames by London Bridge in 1948.

Saint Augustine wrote *De civitate Dei*, in the early fifth century CE, in response to the Visigoths' sacking of Rome. *"On the City of God"* poses the argument of Christianity's superiority over Pagan religions. He, too, describes the Galli removing their manhood, but this time he reports them doing it with their own hands... passing through the streets and alleys of Carthage, with dripping oily hair and [white-] painted faces, with soft limbs and flowing feminine walks, and extracting from merchants the means to continue to live shamefully. He would later describe how Romans believed that by sacrificing their virility, the Galli added to the virile power of Rome.

The second century CE Hellenistic author, Lucian, described the initiation in *De Dea Syria*:[10]

> *While others play the flute and they get into a trance, the young priest gets naked, screams and runs to the middle of the circle of priests, where he grabs a sword and castrates himself immediately. Then he runs through town, holding his manly parts. Then he throws them through a random window and out of that house he shall receive his clothing and jewellery.*

To be clear, Lucian enjoys quite the reputation as a literary wit, so perhaps it might be safer to regard this testimony with suspicion, or caution, at least. It's impossible to gauge the level of its veracity, but as we will see, as we journey through the cults, it was indeed a prerequisite for men to be castrated to become priests of the Mother Goddess, or at least, according to historian Richard Matteoli, circumcised. Some, or at least part of the man's fertility was offered up in sacrifice to The Goddess.[11] To that I shall add, just as a drone bee sacrifices its manhood and his life to his queen.

Cybele, now known as "The Embodiment of Creation, Mother of all Earth, and Creatures in It", arrived in Greece in the fifth century BCE. A temple, *The Metroum*, was dedicated to her as Mother of The Gods in Athens.

The Melissae served alongside the Galli. In *Goddesses and the Divine Feminine: A Western Religious History*, Rosemary Radford Ruether describes how Cybele's traditional rituals began to take on a different shape, adapting to their new culture. *"Nocturnal gatherings of women beating the tympanum and experiencing ecstatic possession"* had found their way to Greece. Cybele was never fully integrated into the Greek religion though, presumably because she shared so many similarities with their own existing Goddesses: Rhea in mainland Greece, Aphrodite on Mount Ida, Artemis in Karia, and Demeter in Samothrake.

However, Rome...

In 204 BCE, Cybele arrived in Rome with great pomp and circumstance after consultations had been made, with both The Oracle of Delphi and the Sibylline Books, about how to overcome threats from Hannibal the Great in The Second Punic War.

Some context is required. The foreshadowing of the tyrant could not have come at a worse time for Rome. Famine and pestilence raged. The threat of war meant the great nation was on the verge of being brought to its knees.

Terrified at the prospects of what might befall them, the Romans leapt at a revelation from The Sibylline Books (a collection of verses from the oracle called The Sybil), that *"if ever a foreign enemy should invade Italy, he could be defeated and driven out if Cybele, the Idaean Mother of the Gods, were brought from Pessinus to Rome."*

It seemed to them that the secret to their success had been revealed and that victory was ordained. Content that they could explain this new arrival by virtue of Rome's supposed Trojan roots, an edict was passed for King Attalus to see if they could procure the sacred rock, Cybele, from Pessinus.

Cybele arrived in Rome, in the form of a meteorite on a most sacred day, the Ides of April (15th), surrounded by all her priests and priestesses. People lined the streets and cheered. The Goddess was met by the emperor, Publius Scipio, and was taken by the women to the Temple of Victory at Palatine, where she was bedecked with flowers. Prayers were offered to her as Magna Mater (Greatest Mother).

Hannibal was subsequently vanquished, and Cybele had secured her place in the heart of Rome.

Cybele had. Her priesthood was not quite as easily accepted.

Their worship was loud, uncouth, and shocking. Their frenzied dances seemed alien to the Romans, and the public castration, well... quite frankly, a disgrace. Romans simply could not tolerate this kind of behaviour, especially since it was forbidden for Romans to be castrated. So, for a while, Roman citizens were banned from becoming priests of Cybele. Later sources confided priests began to keep their bits and relied upon the layers of their floaty frocks to conceal their secret. Naturally, those retaining their members were not allowed to use them.

Now, a new, tamer bee Goddess would take her place. According to Saint Augustine, the Romans worshipped a new bee Goddess, Mellona, *"a Goddess important and powerful regarding bees, taking care of and protecting the sweetness of honey."* Priestesses of Mellona are also thought to have been called Melissa.

Chapter 5

The Bee in Egypt

Indisputably, Apis mellifera has been beloved in the Delta for many a moon, or if not mellifera, some of her cousins, at least. Most probably *Apis mellifera lamarckii*, a smaller and more aggressive insect than the European honey bee.[12]

Even to this day, mud hives travel up and down the River Nile on specially made rafts, moving from one blooming field to the next. As flowers die in one area, they are moved to the next beautiful scape. It has been this way for over five thousand years. The ancient Greeks had great respect for the Egyptians and considered them a holy race. As such, Greek ethos reflects many things they seem to have learnt from the Egyptians. Whilst it would be impossible to visit every area we find correlations between the bee and a creator god, it makes sense to sup just a little nectar from flowers along the Nile.

Honey played a fundamental part in Egypt's life, as tenderly shown in an enchanting set of marriage vows found: "I take thee to wife... and promise to deliver to thee yearly 12 jars of honey." Honey was used for cooking, for healing ailments and wounds, paying taxes, and was also charged as a retinue to be paid by vanquished tribes to their conquerors.

It played a vital part in funerary preparations. Sometimes mummies were embalmed with honey, and bees' wax was used to secure the sarcophagus closed. In the mortuary ritual of the *Opening Of The Mouth*, priests placed honey into the mouth of the Pharaoh's statue. Bees and ritual offerings of honey had relevant connections to the resurrection of the soul.[12]

It seems likely that beekeeping may have been invented by the Egyptians since its most ancient depictions are found in Old Kingdom temples and tombs. Carvings show beekeepers blowing smoke into the hives to calm bees as they remove honeycombs. The temple they are found in, *Shesepibre* (the Delight of Re), dates to around 2450 BCE.

In 1898, archaeologist Ludwig Borchardt discovered the frieze in a room adjacent to the central obelisk, which he called "The Chamber of the Seasons". It is history's earliest representation of beekeeping, showing it in its already advanced form. Each section of the bas-relief details beekeeping activities that occur at specific times of the year.

From left to right there are four scenes:

The beekeeper tends his hives.
Three men pour some honey into earthenware vessels.
The third relief is mostly missing but shows another two men processing the honey.
The honey being sealed into a vessel for storage.[13]

Fascinatingly, the hives used are horizontal tube hives, slightly tapered at the ends. You might find that interesting to remember later when we learn about the Minoan necropolis at Orthi Petra. There are nine horizontal tube hives in total, placed one above the other, probably made of burnt clay. Present-day Egyptian hives still use pipes made of Nile clay and mud.

On the far right, the man extracting honey has something in his hand. Scholars think this might be a small block of dried dung since Egyptian beekeepers still use cow dung to smoke their bees, taking advantage of how slowly and fragrantly it smoulders. Good smoking makes for calm and happy bees. The accompanying hieroglyphs have been translated as "Blowing (or in some translations 'hymning' or smoking), filling, pressing, sealing of honey." Hymning, naturally, might make us think of quietening the bees with song.

The earliest example of the bee symbol also comes from Egypt. Its word is *bjt*. When the kingdoms of Upper and Lower

Egypt were united under one ruler in around 3500 BCE, the bee represented the king of Lower Egypt. He (or She) of the Sedge and Bee. The ruler of Upper Egypt was depicted by a hieroglyph of a reed. The Pharaoh held many titles, one of which was Bee King of "He of The Bee".[12]

From the New Kingdom onwards (c. 1600 BCE), mentions of honey, and depictions of it being made, occur more frequently. The main centre of beekeeping was in Lower Egypt. The bee, who needs water to survive and make honey, relished the rich, lush landscapes along the Nile.

Bees were said to be the tears of Ra, the god believed to rule in all parts of the created world, the Earth, the Sky, and the Underworld. God of the Sun, he was deemed to be the Ruler of Order and All Things Kingly. Legend tells how his tears fell onto the earth and turned into bees. Hence not only bees, but also their wax and honey had originated from the tears of Ra.[13] Documents confirm that the god Amun had an order of priests called *bjty* who were probably the beekeepers who provided honey for temple rituals.

The Temple of Neith at Sais was also referred to as *The House of The Bee*.

Herodotus described Sais (Greek name for the Egyptian city of Sa) detailing it as being an enormous temple complex with connections to a great medical college. Scholars believe the school remained in consistent operation from 3000 BCE-525 BCE. Other sources say it specialised in teaching gynaecology and obstetrics, that it had both female students and faculty members and was run by a woman.

It is suspected, but not proven, that female physician may have been Peseshet, whose name was found during excavations of a tomb in Giza. Born around 2500 BCE, her title was "Lady Overseer of Female Physicians" indicating she supervised a larger contingent of female practitioners and may also have been a clinician, however, that part is uncertain.

Peseshet may be history's earliest woman to have held elevated professional status. She is described as the "King's Associate" and also more solemnly as "overseer of funerary-priests of the king's mother." It is believed she may have graduated over 100 midwives, but this is difficult to prove, since the ancient Egyptian language seems not to have had a specific word for midwife. That they graduate from The House of the Bee *may* dub them Melissae.

These women are referred to in the book of Exodus and while we cannot rely on the Old Testament as being incontrovertible testimony, it does give evidence of their existence at that time.

In Exodus (1:16) we read: *"And he (i.e., the king of Egypt) said: 'When ye do the office of a midwife to the Hebrew women and see them upon the stools...'"*

Excavations uncovered the location of the capital city of Sais in 1993. Evidence shows it had been a busy commercial centre that had traded with many other countries including Syro-Palestine and Greece. It was also discovered they worshiped a local cobra goddess called Wadjet, whose personification can be seen on the Deshret crown of Lower Egypt worn by the goddess, Neith.

Egyptologist Wallis Budge introduces us to Neith from an inscription on a statue of Utchat-Heru, one of her high priests.

She was the first to give birth to anything. She had done so when nothing else had been born. She had never herself been born.

This autogenetic aspect – that she birthed herself from nothing – is seen in both Greek and Latin texts.[14] The celebrated 19th century mystic Mme. Blavatsky relates that Neith is a manifestation of the Vulture Goddess. Blavatsky lists her names as: Neith, Nut, Nepte, Nuk and adds that Neith or Nout is "neither more nor less than Great Mother and yet immaculate virgin, or female God from whom all things proceeded."[15,16]

She is "time without limits."[15,16] As time went by, Neith would also come to be often associated with Ptah-Nun.[15,16]

Creatrix of the creator gods, she is often depicted as veiled, an illusion to the bee's veil-like wings. You might consider how the genus of the bee is hymenopter, and apart from being a woman's intimate membrane, the hymen also depicts the cloth that separates the temple from the Holy of Holies. Naturally, a veil also exists between two worlds.

Plutarch refers to the inscription he saw on her statue in Sais...: "*I am everything that has been, and that is, and that shall be, and no one has ever lifted my garment (peplos)."*

The peplos was a woman's garment. Later we'll discuss how some of the Athenian priestesses were involved in the annual weaving of Athena's peplos. An association exists between Neith and the Greek's Goddess Athena – in fact, many sources describe how Athena *is* Neith.

Egyptian myth places Neith as The Goddess Of Wisdom, The Cosmos, Mothers, Rivers, Water, Childbirth, Hunting, War, Fate and was seen as The Goddess Of Weaving and its original creator.

The Sound of The Bee

In *The Book of Am-Tuat*, the voice of the soul is compared to the buzzing of bees. The book describes the journey the dead Pharoah's soul takes to the underworld. Hourly he is tested for a different secret name he must know, to be able to pass another gate. Therein, he encounters the souls of dead gods, who slumber in a cavern, joined by a long passageway running east to west. Now merged with Osiris, the Pharoah rouses them to rise up onto all fours, to ride with him, in his boat towards the light, their communal voices like "a swarm of bees."[13]

The sanctuary where Osiris was worshiped as God of The Underworld was *Hwt bjt*, the *Mansion of the Bee*.

One epithet Osiris was known by was Osiris Apis.

In this guise, he took on the form of the bull.

Apis was a fertility deity and god of primordial power, who subsequently became associated with the creator god, Ptah. At some point, he must also have developed an association with the bull Goddess Of The Sky, Of Fertility And Women, Hathor. He absorbed her qualities of goodness and bounty, and then further became conflated with the Underworld god, Osiris.

According to Arrian of Nicodemus, Apis was one of the Egyptian gods that Alexander the Great offered sacrifices to when he seized ancient Egypt from the Persians.

It was named Aser-hapi (i.e., **Osiris-Apis**), which then became Serapis, and later was said to represent **Osiris** in his fullness rather than just his Ka – his spirit.

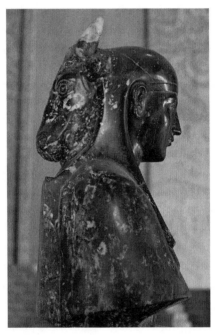

Janiform bust of Antinous as Osiris-Apis (Serapis) springing from a lotus flower. Grey marble, Roman artwork, second part of Hadrian's reign, c. 131-138 CE. Museo Gregoriano Egiziano, Vatican Museums.

The Book of Am-Tuat is an Egyptian cosmological essay that describes the nature of the Tuat, the underworld that the boat of the Sun God, Ra, travels through at night. Ritual prayers in it suggest a person's Ka leaves the body in the form of a bee, and that the afterlife was filled with the sound of humming bees. (Just as Sophocles had said too if you remember: *The swarm of the dead hums…*)

In *Moralia*, Plutarch tells us:

> *The Apis, they say, is the animate image of Osiris, and he comes into being when a fructifying light thrusts forth from the moon and falls upon a cow in her breeding-season.*
>
> *Wherefore there are many things in the Apis that resemble features of the moon, his bright parts being darkened by the shadowy. Moreover, at the time of the new moon in the month of Phamenoth they celebrate a festival to which they give the name of "Osiris' coming to the Moon," and this marks the beginning of the spring. Thus, they make the power of Osiris to be fixed in the Moon, and say that Isis, since she is generation, is associated with him. For this reason, they also call the Moon the mother of the world, and they think that she has a nature both male and female, as she is receptive and made pregnant by the Sun, but she herself in turn emits and disseminates into the air generative principles.* [17]

Phamenoth – the eighth month of the Coptic calendar – lies somewhere between March 10th and April 8th in our Gregorian calendar, depending on the new moon. Interestingly, the actual birthday was memorialised as December 25th, and again, the second coming of Osiris seems to have been celebrated around the spring equinox.

When worshipped in Memphis, the Apis Bull represented maleness and vigour. In life it manifested regeneration through the god Ptah, but in death became Osiris Apis.

The relationship with Ptah is complex. As Dutch archaeologist Henri Frankfort explains

Ptah was never depicted as a bull or believed to be incarnate in a bull; but the Apis bull was called "the living Apis, the herald of Ptah, who carries the truth upwards to him of the lovely face (Ptah)."

In other words, Apis represented the loving vibration that Ptah waited for from man, that sacred intention to connect. Where other gods had their own designated areas of power – Apis was deemed to be infinity itself and the harmonious balance of the universe.

Seen as the divine herald then, there was only ever one Apis Bull at a time. Regarded as sacred, it became quite the mascot, being padded out at religious occasions. Each Apis Bull looked distinctive and almost identical to the others that had gone before it. Chosen from local herds, it was predominately black with various white markings in special places on his body: a triangle on its forehead, a vulture's wing in his back, a crescent moon on its right flank and the mark of a scarab under his tongue. On his tail, he needed to have lustrous double hairs. Oddly, it's almost as if the bull had to have markings that connected him with a drone bee.

Having been identified as the herald, the bull was brought back to the special sanctuary and given a harem of cows. His stall had a window, so you could view him, and when he was paraded about, he was bedecked with ornaments and flowers.

The bull was also deemed to be oracular. Ritually, it was set loose into a special enclosure, with foodstuffs spread around. His movements around the temple were construed as signs, which were then interpreted by priests. His breath was believed to be healing and if he did breathe on you, it was expected that you too may be lucky enough to develop oracular powers. After his prophetic display he was allowed to roam free, and supplicants would bow down before him and pray.

If, and when, the bull reached 25 years old, it was ritually slaughtered and sacrificed, then some of its remains were eaten as sacred food. It was then reputed to have been embalmed and received a sacred funeral, then was buried in a special mausoleum for the bulls, in an enormous granite sarcophagus, under the temple of Serapis at Saqqara. Any calves it had sired were likewise slaughtered, embalmed and buried. Its mother previously having been slaughtered and dedicated to Isis.

In *The Sacred Bee* Hilda Ransome describes a slightly different version of events:

> *the females, who are sacred to Isis, are thrown into the river (Nile), but the males are buried in the suburbs of the towns with one or both of their horns appearing above the surface of the ground to mark the place. When the bodies are decayed a boat comes, at an appointed time, from the island of Prosopitis, which is a portion of the Delta, and calls at the various cities in turn to collect the bones of the oxen.*

This seems more likely to be true to me because in a YouTube video by "Igor Travels The World" about The Serapeum, the unnamed guide describes how he had read in a book that one of the mummified bulls could be found in the agricultural museum, which he visited, found the bull, and discovered that, rather than being mummified, the remains were a skeleton.[18]

Serapis becomes important to us later in the book, since he, like the Greek god Asclepius, was associated with the dream incubation of the Melissae priestesses. When the amalgamation of Greco and Egyptian religions started to take place, the Apis took on the Hellenistic fashion of being depicted as a man. Worship of Serapis was only prevalent for around a century which may have been Egyptian annoyance at one of their gods being made to look so Greek! In illustrations, he is depicted with a beard and masses of curls. Serapis is the anthropomorphic expression of the Apis Bull.

So where, I wonder, does Apis come into it?

Because Apis is the Latin word for bee, but this one is a bull. Antigonos of Carystus wrote, in the second century BCE, that in *"Egypt if you bury the ox in certain places,"* the result was that *"bees fly out; for the ox putrifies and is resolved into bees."* Virgil expresses this same belief and it is also told by Varro, Ovid, and Pliny. Indeed, the expressions *"bugenès melissae"* and *"taurigenae apes"* meant *"oxen-born bees"* and the ancient Greeks occasionally referred to honey bees as *"bugenès"* or *"taurigenae".*[19]

The bull was a key sacramental creature, particularly in the Minoan culture in Crete which we explore later. In "Virgil and the Bees: A study in Ancient Apicultural Lore", B.G. Whitfield described how a ritual of "closing of the ears and nostrils of the beast seem[ed] to have as an aim the preservation of the soul within the carcass". Somehow, the bull's essence was then believed to be captured within the bees. The bees were the soul of the bull, and the bull was Osiris, and later in Greece, the mighty Zeus.[20] Again, we get this feeling of inextricable connection between milk and honey.[20,21] Bees were the bringers of new souls, and many souls would be born into the world from Apis.

We should remember Osiris is not the god of regeneration; Ptah is, and indeed so was Isis. Osiris is **resurrection**, a process that could only be brought about through observance of dedicated rituals for the gods.

Porphyry said:

All souls, however, proceeding into generation, are not simply called bees, but those who live justly, and who, having performed such things as are acceptable to the gods, will return whence they came. For this insect loves to return to the place whence it came and is eminently just and sober.

The bee and cow are linked, perhaps in the same way as milk and honey.

Chapter 6

The Bee Goddess Reaches Greece

The Greek bee priestesses are thought to have been directly influenced by the Minoan culture that developed in Crete around 3000 BCE, and indeed much of our most beautiful imagery comes from there. This is explored separately in Chapter 17 when we understand the bee allegory better.

For now, we'll focus on mainland Greece.

The Greek Dark Ages (c. 1200 BCE-700 BCE) was a time of tribal communities, each with its own mysterious canon of beliefs. Although "pagan" means polytheistic (many gods) – its literal translation comes from the Latin word *paganus*, which means rural, of the countryside, rustic or local.

Each tribe revered their own local mysterious, wonderful, and terrifying entities.

Unlike today's religions, they had no set texts framing their belief systems. Dogma was superfluous, since religion played out in what they observed around them. Fascination with the Earth informed their rituals and stories.

Deities, nature spirits, water sylphs, nymphs, devas, creatures...

Sacred places, magic trees, spirit dwellings, caves, mountain tops, springs, forests, delves...

Things that protected and seemed to speak.

Then around the eighth century BCE, Greece started to change, becoming orientalised.[22] Ships from Mongolia, Siberia, and even further into Asia and China, moored in the ports of the Greek islands, laden with glorious fabrics and spices. Along with precious cargos, merchants brought shamanistic tales and Archaic Greece saw an explosion of technology, art, and poetry.

Scholars Walter Burkert and Martin Litchfield West are convinced that tales from Mesopotamia and Phoenicia heavily influenced the Greek religion of the Archaic Period. Homer's *Odyssey*, according to Burkert, was directly inspired by the Babylonian *Epic of Gilgamesh* and West argues that Hesiod's *Theogony* and *Cosmogony* are Grecian versions of Phoenician myths.

The Bible called the Phoenicians, Canaanites. Those of the Land of Milk and Honey.

The Archaic Period was a time of massive cultural, philosophical, and political growth. It marked the beginning of the Hellenistic fascination with rebirth,[23] and is also believed to be when the City State, the *polis*, came into being.

Still today, Athens is recognised as the foundation stone of democracy. The polis stood at its core and was founded entirely upon the wisdom of the hive. The democracy of Athens was based on a communal imagining of not just living *with* the animal kingdom, but as if they *were* bees and other insects.

The polis mirrored how bees live in colonies and are subject to an irresistible urge to create. They build comb, manage their nursery, tend nymphs, bring pollen, water, and nectar into the hive. They manufacture antibiotic fortifications for the hive – *propolis* – note that even the name means *For The City State* in this context. Importantly, they do it despite the fact they will never enjoy the bounty themselves. Their short lives mean these services are entirely selfless acts.

A bee's capacity to manufacture honey was conceived to be both miraculous and divine – a kind of natural alchemy, and ancient European beekeepers believed virtue to be paramount for its creation. If the keeper didn't display honesty or goodness, then bees would simply not produce honey for them.

Those last two paragraphs deserve full consideration, because perhaps more than anything you will read in this book, they tell you much about how these bee priestesses were perceived.

Just like the hive, the polis was seen as a single organism, always working for the good of the collective. To them, bees symbolized diligence, industry, and obedience to competent leaders. The religious and political nature of the polis – being formed of many smaller units all fitting seamlessly together – seemed to them, to be like a honeycomb. Each person residing within the unit was expected to perform his or her function effortlessly, and without question, for the good of the hive, in irresistible service to The Goddess.

Thus, citizens of the polis were bees; priestesses were bees, and the goddess controlling and narrating the story, who bestowed favour and bounty upon her society, was the bee deva.

Interestingly though, Aristotle described the Greek belief of a Bee *King* ruling the hive whom he related as being clearly superior. Whilst he does not elucidate what exactly he bases this notion of superiority upon, he described the king as being larger and longer than his compatriots in the hive.

In *The Honey Bee and Apian Imagery in Classical Literature*, Doctor of Philosophy, Rachel Carson, points out how Aristotle seems to be exaggerating here, perhaps in an attempt to make the king seem even more superior than he actually was. The queen bee – as we now recognise her to be – is distinguishable as being bigger than the rest of her hive, but the task of identifying the shy queen, who prefers to stay in the dark, is difficult enough, that some modern beekeepers choose to mark her with a coloured dot to keep tabs on where she goes.[24]

Presumably, the more they stared into the hive and watched what the bees were up to, the more epiphanies they experienced about the mysteries of life.

In *The Greeks and the Irrational*, historian and psychic E.R. Dodds describes how, around the fifth century BCE, the Greek culture seems to have experienced a bit of a wobble, where they began to question their shamanistic practices. But, rationality didn't last long and soon enough, we see the religion begin to evolve again but this time growing and beginning to merge with more Eastern philosophies. Now it began to encompass astrology, alchemy, and wizardly medicines.[23]

"Rationality didn't last long..."

What do we mean by that? Because even as I write it, it feels rather patronising, but that's a symptom of looking through those modern-day glasses Sourvinou-Inwood warned us about wearing, because the temptation is to imagine Greece as being somewhat Western, but as we've seen, actually their influences came from the East. Much of the political, the philosophical and even the scientific thinking displays cultural overtones from Egypt, Mesopotamia and even India.[25]

If we're not careful, we fall into the trap of imagining an Apollonian world, when actually their belief system was more Dionysian.[26] This is an important distinction. What does it mean?

Apollo and Dionysos were brothers and sons of Zeus.

Apollo was the God of the Sun. He rules rational thinking and order. The world that you and I presently live in likes to order things, categorise, and make sense of them.

That's Apollonian.

It's logic, prudence, and purity. With that, we accept the idea that logic can be conceptualised as being within the limits of our consciousness, and that which is experienced within the neat fields of time and space. Ideas within this Apollonian framework fit tidily into terms of opposites: light, dark, male, female, possible and impossible.

But just like any other family, the contrasts between siblings could not be more different. It should be the qualities of Apollo's more ecstatic brother, Dionysos, that colour our imaginings of Greece.

The androgynous god of wine and dance, Dionysos rules irrationality, debauchery, and chaos. He is the god of ecstasy, transgression, transformation, and excess.[27]

His cult is "of the souls".

A potted version of some of his Orphic beliefs is a person was born with Dionysian perfectly pure spirit, housed in evil, chaotic Titanic flesh. Spirits were believed to drift down from the Heavens, disturbed by the chaos of creation, moving around on the breeze, accompanied by the bees, until children were born. At that moment, the bees then accompanied the Dionysian spirit down to Earth, where it was breathed into the body at a baby's first gasp.

The Orphic Mysteries viewed the body as the spirit's tomb, fated to exist on the Wheel of Birth – to be born, live, die, and then to be reincarnated for up to 10,000 years. The soul's journey was influenced by good deeds and bad. Today, we might say it's reminiscent of Hinduism (and, indeed, the Hindu Sadhus do worship the Lord Dionysos as bringer of their monsoon), but this belief of reincarnation originated in Greece in the sixth century BCE and then perhaps influenced the contemporaneous Upanishads who introduced ideas of regeneration and karma to India.

Dionysos' devotees, the Maenads, revelled in the god's world of wine and madness, their long, loose hair wild around their faces as they danced his orgiastic praise. In Euripides' play, *The Bacchae*, we hear of a terrified man's horror at having accidentally stumbled upon a secret maenadic rite in the forest. Panic-stricken, he describes women with snakes in their hair, suckling wolves at their breasts with honey oozing from their staffs. Their *thyrsus* staffs, fennel stalks topped with pinecones, symbolise Dionysos' fertility and the spreading of his seed, but also the irrational flow of nature. Ivy, the keeper of liminal knowledge, snakes around the stem. *(Fig. 6a)* It was said the pinecone was wrapped with a strap and emitted a humming sound when twizzled.[28]

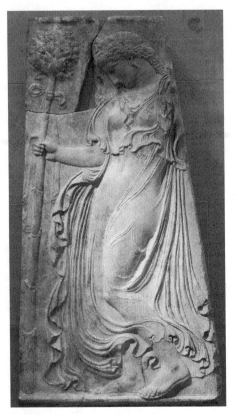

Dancing Maenad Roman copy of Greek original attributed to Kallimachos, c. 425-400 BCE, at the Metropolitan Museum of Art.

The dead are fed through their blood offerings. Their dresses flow free, weighted by animal skins that drape from their shoulders, trophies of leopards ripped apart as they've despatched them from gateways to places that are "other". (Whether that ripping is literal or symbolic is not clear.)

The great power symbol of female knowledge, the snake, sits atop their heads, in testimony of the numinous. Ready to whisper insights of intuition, the serpent is keeper of sacred knowledge including that undiscovered wisdom of medicine and science.

Dionysos acts as medium between the living and the dead.

His realm is that of emotions and instincts, and those places within us that are wild. It is he who shatters, in order to bring forth new creativity. Whenever he appears in myths, he bursts in, with great disruption. He obliterates anything settled in his path. Creativity is essentially a "breaking down" business, an opportunity to disrupt and start again. Thus, Dionysos shatters consciousness, so that psyche can be re-membered. We should comprehend by his chaotic state then that he, by definition, *cannot* be defined by anything as linear as time and space.

Dionysos was the German philosopher Friedrich Nietzsche's favourite god; he believed that our modern-day overly sanitised Apollonian existence lacks the vitality of the Dionysian Tragic Outlook, which pervaded the ancient Greek world. Dionysos, from his very conception, had endured dreadful loss and had continued to do so through his existence. And yet, quite marvellously and inspirationally, he continued to revel in life's eternal fest.

It's in the process of bearing the weight of nihilism, Nietzsche says, of plunging into the depths of sorrow and fully experiencing the desperation that everything is most certainly lost, and somehow simultaneously soaring upon thermals of great joy, that we fully embrace life. Consider, then, how the role of the priestess played out, that she would experience, and by extension, her students would be encouraged to experience life in its most vibrant of colours. Indeed, reflect on how the honey bee lands on each flower, ecstatically revelling in her feast of different pollens, regardless of what sort of pollen she finds.

Perhaps the greatest aid to imagining these women's world is to learn that one out of every three infants is believed to have died in the first years of its life. Can you imagine the collective grief of the nation? And yet somehow it did not cripple them.

To be a celebrant of Dionysos demanded you learn to feel the exquisite rawness of life and relish every moment of it, dancing naked through the trees, fully comprehending that there are no explanations for life's torture. Celebrating the liberation that bitter experience always defies logic and thus explanation.

Chapter 7

The Life Time of The Ancient Greek Priestess

I've discussed this research with many women, and the response has been a resoundingly startled silence and then similar comebacks every time. "So, these Greek women weren't silent and locked away at home then?"

Maybe. I'm undecided, and of course we have no real way of knowing.

But, you know, it doesn't feel like they *could* have been, to me. The opposite, in fact. To me, they seem to have been powerfully emancipated people.

As far as I can see, ancient Greek women lived rich and vibrant social lives directed through religious function. Clearly, not all of them were priestesses, but those who were, had the capacity to climb to the high ranks of their profession that were at least equal to priests. While not directly engaged in political function, religion was so closely entwined with politics that consulting the priestess about decisions of state was not only deemed to be acceptable, but it also seems to have been commonplace.

Melissa's role as a Grecian woman was to thank The Goddess for *all* aspects of her being. Since each Goddess looked after a different dimension, prayers and sacrifices also needed to be offered to several deities too. To Athena for her wisdom, Aphrodite for her sensuality. Gratitude was given to Artemis for care before marriage. Hera protected the heroes and Tyche was the benefactor of good chance. Demeter must be praised and placated for the harvest and the Queen of the Underworld, Persephone, was to be graced if one was to hope for her to intervene after death on your behalf.

And we haven't even thought about the gods here.

The Attic calendar follows the changing of the seasons, starting and ending on the summer solstice new moon. The climax of the Athenian year was the Eleusinian Mysteries, a once-in-a-lifetime occasion for which people travelled from right across the ancient world to participate. The Greater Mysteries was a nine-day festival which took place in the autumn. Initiates had to have undertaken the five-day Lesser Mysteries, the previous spring, to take part. These were just two of Demeter's *seven* festivals. Seen in that light, you can see that being a supplicant in the Greek religion gave women ample chance to socialise, although The Mysteries were somewhat unusual since both men and women could attend. For the most part, festivals were only open to one or other sex. In Demeter's cult, for example, Thesmophoria was only available to women.

At these gatherings, women socialised with others of a similar age. They chatted about their health, listened to each other's moans about marriage and celebrated the landmarks of their age. It must have been an incredibly healing bond against loneliness and the everyday challenges that gender differences bring. Together they expressed their personal changes against the ritual calendar.

Weekends did not exist in ancient Greece. Rituals punctuated their calendar giving it structure and meaning. There was no single agreement on what happened when; each district observing its own calendar. Some began on the winter solstice, but the Athenian Attic Calendar aligned with the summer one. It included 140 state days, and 180 religious days, demonstrating the larger emphasis the Athenians placed on religion.

For that, women had a vital part to play.

Grecian cults chose deity representatives in their likenesses. For the most part, men served gods and women served their

Goddesses. There are exceptions that disprove the rule, such as the cult of Hekate where the highest official was a priest, but in a pantheon of male and female deities then, at least half the jobs belonged to women.

In *Portrait of a Priestess*, Breton Connelly describes 150 ancient Greek priestesses whose names have been discovered through a variety of means. Some are from names carved into statues or onto their bases, which betrays much about their status. Only the names of priestesses and victorious warriors were allowed to be inscribed onto portrait statues. That we can still find them today shows how specially the priestess was set apart. Some names have also been found in tomb inscriptions, and in some cases their names are written into historical record.

Empty words though; these names offer us nothing of substance about who these women were, what they did, or even what they were for.

In some ways, art helps, but the stories it can tell are limited. If we look at a vase, for example, it can show us what women looked like and some of the things they got up to as they celebrated. In the same way, if we consider the context an object might have been used in, it offers clues into what the woman's role might have been. A depiction on a wine jug probably has different significance to one found on a funeral vase, for example.

The problem is though, when we look at a woman in an illustration, we can't really be sure who we are seeing. She might be a priestess, it might be a depiction of a Goddess, or even a mythical representation from antiquity. She might even be just your average housewife, carrying out her duties to a goddess.

One of the most common illustrations we will see is of women using the *oinochoē* (jug) and *philae* (bowl).

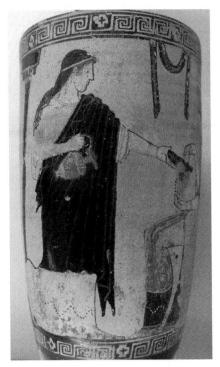

Woman offering libations. The temple columns may depict her as a priestess. British Museum. Photograph by Marie-Lan Nguyen.

The jug and bowl were used as a sacred pair. If you see them together, you can almost certainly assume it depicts a ritual. A libation was poured from the jug into the bowl and was then poured onto the altar for the goddess. The offerings, usually in the form of wine or mead, but perhaps in grain form such as barley, were offered in grateful thanks and homage to the deities for all their favours, or in memory of the dead.

As the libation hit the flames, the blaze roared as the goddess showed her pleasure.

Just as incense carried *Aeros* – the loving intentions – of the supplicant (the worshipper), pouring libations invited the goddess to take control of proceedings. It served to reassure the supplicant that the occasion had the deity's blessing. Surely, that meant the sacred encounter would commence without a hitch.

The verb *spendō* (σπένδω), to pour a libation, also translates to *conclude a pact*. Quite literally, the pouring of a libation meant security to the Greeks, an insurance policy, if you will. On accepting the libation, the gods were called upon to guarantee their best efforts to deliver their end of the bargain.

Since libations generally accompanied prayer, wine would be poured onto sacrificed meat before it was placed onto the altar, then again on the ashes when it had burned.

The Greeks prayed by raising their hands skyward, or extending their libation bowl, but if the offering were to a chthonic deity (of the underworld: such as Demeter or Persephone), offerings would be poured onto the ground, instead of the altar, before anyone could take their first swig. First sup always went to the divine guest of honour.

In a ritual setting, this was done by the priestess, but offering libations was one of the most common methods of worship in ancient Greece. Women were allowed to offer their own libations to The Goddess, and it's likely that pious women performed private rites at the family's morning and evening meals. Given that, then, we cannot assume characters holding a jug and bowl are always priestesses.

To us, a vase, is a vase, is a vase, but to bring the priestess to life, her image must be seen in context, through the eyes of the woman who, two thousand years ago, held it in her hands.

One reliable way to tell whether we can say a woman depicted on a vase, or piece of art, is a priestess, is whether she holds the temple key. An enormous, long pole, the key turned at right angles, and right angles again, then hooked into leather straps on the other side of the door, to slide the bolt across to gain access to the sanctuary. (The key only became a commonplace depiction from the fifth century BCE.)

To become keeper of the key was an enormous responsibility since the temple sanctuary housed tremendous wealth. The priestess would rise early in the morning, purify herself through washing and then go and open the temple.

Another fairly stable symbol is a pair of columns framing her on either side, placing her in an illustration of a temple. There she would light the altar fire and draw the goddess into the space.

The only person allowed into the sacred space, with the goddess' statue, it was the priestess' job to keep it clean. When asked to by supplicants, she would draw back the curtain to the idol, lay down sacrifices and ask favours from the goddess in prayer.

She poured libations, and before prayers could take place, the supplicant had to be purified through washing, and to be cleansed with the winnowing sieve.

Whilst the function of the priestess was to act as intermediary between woman and goddess, in service to the deity, it behoves us to consider her role as far more complex than that.

Inscriptions bear testimony to the levels of dedication and financial commitment that priestesses gave to their roles and the great privileges they enjoyed in return.

An inscription on a pedestal that graced the statues of a priestess named Epigone and her husband was found in Mantineia, Greece. Dating back to the first century BCE, it describes her as being "respectable and husband loving", extolling her virtues as a benefactor.

It reads, *"Sparing no expense, she piously honoured the gods and lavishly feasted the populace."*

Breton Connelly relates how, with the support of her husband, Epigone's priestess career built a lavish marketplace with a covered hall, porticoes and banquet rooms complete with heating. She filled it with all manner of treasures and generally made the city of Mantineia a lovelier place to live.

It's not clear how much a priestess depended on her husband's income, but it is obvious the Melissae were women of power and significant independent means. Mandatory fees were paid to the priestess for her help in offering sacrifices on one's behalf, and she was also entitled to take home a portion of every sacrifice she presided in.

The function of the priestess was to grow the cult, to produce prosperous festivals, and to ensure the community thrived within the bounds of a successful contract with the deity. Prayers were offered in a manner pleasing to the goddess, overseen by the ritual of the priestess and her enforcement of sacred law.

Priestesses usually came from high-born families and specific tribes. Marriages between the most prominent tribes strengthened the priestly classes, and it is not unusual to find a husband, wife and children all serving within the temple.

Bees, Bears, Doves, and Foals

Not all Melissae were priestesses, and not every priestess was known as Melissa. Likewise, contrary to what herbal texts would have us believe, they were not only affiliated to Demeter, or indeed only to Greece, being found much further afield in Asia Minor and Egypt for instance. They belonged to a tradition that had originated from many thousands of years before.

The term Melissa gives us three pointers:

Firstly, it tells us something about the goddess she served.

For example: Aphrodite's priestesses were called Doves, the *arktoi*, or Bears, were the representatives of Artemis at Brauron (also known as Vrauron), and *poloi* – the Foals – were celebrants of Dionysos at Leukippides at Sparta.

The Melissae, or bees, celebrated various aspects of the fertility goddess. As we have seen, they celebrated Demeter – Kore (the correct name for the cult of Demeter and her daughter, Persephone) in Athens, but Melissae also worshipped Artemis of Ephesos, Cybele, Rhea, Aphrodite, and Dionysos too.[29]

Each of these female deities is recognised as **Bee Goddess** and is termed Melissa just as the priestesses were. By extension we can now also say the priestesses worshipped goddesses who were not necessarily bees, but were also associated with the moon, namely Hekate, for example. Further, some of the Melissae were oracles.

The second point we might be able to infer is that a priestess' cultic name may also hint to some aspect of the activity within that cultus.

Small two-handled cups, known as a *krateriskoi* found at Brauron (where the "bears" were, remember?), show images of lines of naked, young girls with their arms outstretched, holding wreaths. Behind a palm tree, is depicted a bear, lurking, and the girls look afraid, as if they are being chased.

It seems reasonable to assume this might depict a ritual where young daughters of Athenians play the "Arkteia" – that is the "Running From the Bear." But we should exercise caution. Are we seeing an ancient Greek scene, or a mythical representation drawn from antiquity?

Either way, it suggests that a bear, or perhaps someone *mimicking* a bear, might have played a part in this ritual dedicated to Artemis. Thus, if a priestess is listed as being involved in the cult of Demeter, we might be able to infer that something to do with their cultic activity may have an association with bees.

Depending on which cult she celebrated, we may be able to infer some inkling about her age. The priestess of Demeter Kore was an adult, married woman, of childbearing age, with the notable exceptions of priestesses of Demeter Chthonia who were drawn from post-menopausal crones.

Lastly, if age and geography allowed, theoretically it could be possible for a Melissa to also be a dove or a bear. That is to say: she was not restricted to just one cult and can often be seen in inscriptions, as having served more than one goddess in her lifetime.

Historians mention a specific type of Melissa being at the rituals of Eleusis called *Panageis* (Holy Ones or often simply translated as Bees), who have been described by modern commentators as being celibate auxiliaries. However, this would be at odds with the standard description of Demeter's Melissae as married women.

Buildings in the temple complexes are sometimes also referred to as panageis, so it could be that the name may have been given to priestesses who had undergone purification through a period of celibacy prior to the ritual in these places where they went to be set apart for a while. Ordinary celebrants at Demeter's celebrations of Thesmophoria are also termed Melissa, so to me, at least, it seems likely that the Panageis were the most highly developed Melissa priestesses, but it's impossible to know. Perhaps, by the end of the book, you will have your own thoughts about this.

There has been much speculation as to what the Melissae priestesses' duties may have been, but they remain unknown. It's thought they were ministers and that they may have been the only ones allowed to touch the Eleusinian *hiera* – the sacred objects – but this is entirely conjecture.

Cult Agent

At the surface level, the role of the priestess was an extension of her household duties. Just as she cared for her husband and home, she cared for the sanctuary she was servant of, its idols, and by extension, the goddess. She would keep the deity image clean, light the altar fire, and ensure people offering prayers looked the part.

It is difficult to reconstruct a set dress code for what they should or shouldn't have looked like, since each cult had their own locally ordained rules. However, we do know that certain colours were frowned upon as being ostentatious to The Goddess while others seem to have been promoted.

One sacred law from the sanctuary of *Demeter Thesmophoros*, in Arkadia, dated fifth century BCE, forbade worshippers from wearing gold or purple. No face powder was to be worn or fancy dresses. Any frocks worn with decoration on must be subsequently sacrificed to the goddess.

In contrast, the Eleusinian priesthood wore purple cloaks called *phoinikis*. Later, we'll hear how initiates of The Mysteries were sworn to secrecy, but when a man named Andokides was found guilty of parodying the ritual at somebody's dinner party, the priests and priestesses ominously shook "their purple cloaks" at him for breaking the sacred vow, a crime punishable by death.

Purple fabric was treasured and prohibitively expensive to buy, since the dye was manufactured through a lengthy and rigorous process involving ground seashells. Anyone dressing in gold or purple subliminally boasted high worth. One legend tells how the High Priest of Eleusis wore his finery to head into the Battle of Marathon. When he was taken prisoner, the enemy took one look at his dress and concluded they must have captured the king. Outlawing opulence levelled status. Only the Eleusinian officials were elevated. Purple made them stand out. Interestingly too, bees can see very few colours, and purple is proven to be their favourite.

Beneath the purple cloak, sacred law demanded Melissae, and other female officials at Eleusis, wore long tunics with fringes at the bottom, or tunics with no coloured borders. We know this undergarment as the *chiton*.

Ironically, since statues of women could only be of priestesses or goddesses, arguably it may be that we know more about what priestesses wore than ordinary women. They show the chiton tied under the bust, with a sash or *himation* draped over it.

The himation should cost no more than two minas, which was no modest amount of money. In 2015, it was calculated that a drachma was equal to around $25, and there were 100 drachmae to a mina. Either clothes were incredibly expensive, or people *really* dressed up to go to temple.

If someone turned up to offer sacrifices but didn't meet the priestess' exacting standards for appearance, they could be turned away, or even cursed. Sacred laws belonged to the sanctuary and were enforceable through law by the priestess.

Breton Connelly also relates that it was forbidden for supplicants to wear cosmetics or perfume when they entered the Temple.

Greek ritual dance expert Laura Shannon tells us:

The word kósmos (κόσμος) gives us the word kósmima (κόσμημα), jewellery – silver and gold like the moon and sun, with glinting gems like the stars and planets – as well as the word kosmitiká (κοσμητικά), cosmetics. These adornments were used by priestesses in classical Greece, not to emphasise their individual beauty, but rather to identify them in their public role as instruments of cosmic beauty, harmony, and order.[30]

It was intentional that the priestess looked different to the rest of the women; that she stood out.

Scent has a primary part to play in the Melissa cognisance. Bees are deaf, and have limited vision, but their lives are driven by vibration, taste, and fragrance. The same becomes true of the Melissa priestess. From the malty scent of baking bread to the stench of the farmyard, common smells ritualistically repeated religious experiences. They were common markers that reminded the supplicants of all the places deities could be.

I believe *kosmitiká* also encompasses the idea of perfume, not least because scent contributes so profoundly to a person's perception of the situation that they find themselves in. That's the very point of incense, surely, and indeed of an anointing oil?

Consider that, there were clear associations with the idea of bees; that the *polis* was a hive, and thus its female citizens were workers. At rituals, they made and ate [bee] bread, smoked the altar, feasted on honey...

The bees' ritual space *must* have smelt of Melissa. I recently moved my own bees from a tatty old hive to a beautiful one The Silent One made, and next day it reeked of the Nasonov they had secreted to reassure the colony.

I like to imagine priestesses circulating amongst the workers, distributing the scent of Nasonov, assuring everyone the hive was queenright, that The Goddess was in residence doing everything they needed her to do.

Every ritual was carefully choreographed to give a particular, memorable, impression, and at every point we are supposed to remember that the priestesses are bees. The most persuasive way to do that would be through sensory association. To me, it seems to be the fragrant link that completes the illusion.

All through Greek literature we hear how beautiful the goddesses were imagined to be, and it seems priestesses were selected for their loveliness too.

Likewise, Aphrodite in her allure and Persephone in her darkness as Queen of The Underworld were reflected in the looks of women chosen to portray them. Long lustrous locks, dark hair for Persephone and golden barley-coloured tresses for Demeter.

The following excerpt, written in the third century CE, by Xenophon of Ephesos, gives us a glimpse into how the priestess might have been seen as she passed by the crowds in procession.

A prodigy of loveliness (who) far surpassed all the other maidens. Her eyes were shining sometimes like a girl's and sometimes severe as a chaste Goddess. Her dress was a frock of purple, her wrap a fawn skin and a quiver hung down by her shoulders. She carried a bow and a javelin and dogs fled at her heels. Time and again the Ephesians saw her in the sacred procession and bowed down as to Artemis... some of the spectators asserted that she was the very Goddess and others declared she was replica fashioned by The Goddess.

(An Ephesian Tale 1.2.5-7)

There was a requirement of "being whole" to be a member of the priesthood, which had originally suggested to me they had to be virgins, but that was a wrong turn on my part – we'll investigate the issue of virginity later.

Actually, it was physical defects that were deal breakers for entering office, and in later periods when priesthoods began to be bought and sold, adverts insisted the new person in office must be "Healthy and Whole."

When someone was accepted into post, one of the "interview" requirements was to be inspected to ensure they were blemish free and well enough to serve. I understand that, even today, should a Greek Orthodox priest be unlucky enough to lose a finger, he must still ask for a special dispensation to keep his job. After my adventures in the bee kingdom, I suspect the term probably alluded to a robust mental stability too.

In death, the priestess was buried with her regalia. The gold death mask of the wife of a Bottiaean ruler and High Priestess known as the Lady of Archontiko has been found, dating to 540 BCE.

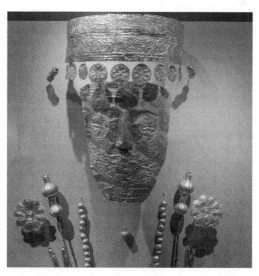

Funerary Mask of Lady of Archontiko. Photograph by Egisto Sani.

She served as mediator of divine blessings for her community of Archontiko northwest of Pella, near Thessaly. The cemetery where she was discovered had nearly 1000 graves of varying wealth and status. Her grave (No. 458) was excavated in the most elite section of the western cemetery, in the same burial cluster as some of the community's warriors.

She is veiled, held in darkness. Not to keep the outside world out, but to keep The Goddess in.[31]

Women's Roles in the Religion

As Melissae priestesses, the women learnt to mirror many aspects of roles played out in the hive. Depending on the type of priestess she was, she may have been oracle, soul midwife, dream weaver, weather priestess, guardian of the crops or fertility matron. Through time, and careful meditation, the women transformed the energetic imprints of their wombs into shapeshifting spaces, which they used as bays of oracular knowing and connections to star realms.

Through focused intent, they learnt to control their inner necktaries (energy centres), how to use and control their internal fluids and energy systems, not only to heal themselves, but also to connect and communicate with other dimensions, whether that be on the cosmic level, or through nature, sound, scent, or colour.

Using these extraordinary skills, it was their job to bring and retain World order, through ritual, through healing of people and the Earth, through divination and oracles.

The greatest and most powerful of the priestesses was the representative of Athena Polias, the patron deity of Athens. Realistically though, this was available to only a very narrow margin of women since inscriptions on statues and tombstones seem to suggest this position tended to be filled by women of one particular tribe. Of the priestesses listed from the end of the fifth century BCE to the second century CE, 25 of the roles were held by women of the Eteoboutadae clan.

The clan claimed to be one of Athens' founding families. Holding the position of High Priestess of Athena Polias brought great prominence to their households. The incarnation of Athena, as protector of the polis, the High Priestess wielded enormous religious and political influence.

We should exercise caution though. Because this familial connection perhaps implies an easy nepotism to gain a role. However, the reverse may be true. In today's vocabulary the term high priestess suggests a higher rank, a manager maybe, but it seems unlikely that any such hierarchy existed. The term high priestess does indeed allude to sovereignty, but more than any kind of seniority as we might imagine it, it speaks of mastery of her craft.

The term "high priestess" referred to one who has passed through several levels of initiations and elevations. It pertained to their function within the temple tradition and how active they were within it. How many temple duties did they perform, how many rituals or circles did they conduct, and how many students were in their care?

My own High Priestess reminded me that neither is there a hierarchy within the hive.[32] We call her the Queen, but she is the sexual servant and the egg layer, committing herself to solitude in the darkness, surrounded by sisters who are differently free. She works in absolute service to the hive. Her life is a devotion to those whom she loves.[32] The role of the high priestess had nothing to do with self-elevation or aggrandizement (which must have been incredibly difficult for the women of antiquity given their wealth and status); her function is service, not self-gain.[33]

In Pliny's work *On Natural History*, he writes of one High Priestess of Athena Polias, Lysimache, who served for 64 years. Her statue had been carved by Demitrios, a sculptor well respected for his skill in creating true likenesses of his subjects and who had flourished around 350-400 BCE.

The marble base that supported her bronze statue has since been found, near the south wall of the Acropolis, close to Athena's temple, the Parthenon.

The inscription is damaged and both the priestess' and sculptor's names were missing but scholars now feel confident that Pliny had read the same plaque and remembered the famous woman nearly five hundred years later.

It reads:

[Lysimache], daughter of Drakontes and lived for eighty-four years.
[In all for six]ty four years [she served] Athena and saw four generations of children.
[Lysimache,] mother of [---]es of Phyla
[Demitrios] made [the statue]

It is known that Lysimache had a prominent brother, Lysikles, who served as secretary of the treasury from 416/415 BC. It could be that Lysikles exerted influence to secure such an illustrious role for Lysimache, but we don't know. The inscription bears witness to the fact that rather than being the virginal priestess we might have come to expect, Lysimache had married, borne children and seemingly retained her priesthood long after her fertility had left her.

Lysimache's role was seemingly permanent, but not all high priesthoods were. What should be stressed though, is that a priestess seems only to have ever served one Goddess at a time. Her dedication to the divinity was deemed to be a total act, however, their service might be temporary or seasonal, depending on the ritual structure of the sanctuary they worked in. With my ex-recruitment consultant head on, that might imply a hidden path of priestesshoods serving as stepping stones of experience, but if it is there, I cannot see any obvious evidence.

Next in the ranking of the priesthoods, after the priestess of Athena Polias came our Melissa, the Priestess of Demeter.

It's clear that girls from prominent families entered the cult early, taking on simple roles, gradually moving up through a variety of positions that matched their age and status.

Both the offices of Demeter Kore at Eleusis and Athena Polias were *eponymous titles*. This means dates in history were marked by the tenure of their priesthood. Their names were inscribed onto the bases of their statues and were held up for all history to remember.

In death, the priestess marks the times things took place, and in life, it was the priestess' presence that made space sacred. Her role in space is fascinating.

Greece's Classical Period was known as the age of music and dance; rhythm and chorus stood at the heart of their religion. Different to how we recognise chorus today, music encompassed rhythm, music, song, movement, but also the space set aside for it. Where it was performed, and the context it was perceived in, was extremely important.

The idea of space is quite different to the way we perceive it today.

Where you and I might have a disagreement with our neighbour, about where the boundary of our property is, we can usually resolve it by looking at title deeds and comparing the physical landscape to maps. No boundary distinctions existed in the polis. After all, this is a hive, remember. Everything belongs to the colony.

Today, we might have a few public buildings, but the majority of our buildings are residential. In Greece, enormous communal centres formed the heart of the polis with residential buildings scattered round.

If you purchased a property, you claimed the space by offering a sacrifice. But, by virtue of the sacrifice having been made within a communal space, it too belonged to the community.

Processions, headed up by basket carrying priestesses called *kanephoros*, delineated sacred space. The kanephoroi carried the *hiera* (sacred things) in baskets on their heads. Journeying between the city and sacred spaces, informed special associations between places. In turn, the presence of the priestess sanctified the journey to a deeper, more hallowed space. On Monday they may have walked past the Acropolis to get groceries, for example, but on Tuesday, escorted by a priestess, meant the street now became a hallowed space. Nestled in the beautiful golden rocks, Athens was always beautiful, but when the priestess was near, it became wondrous.

Where the priestess designated the space as sacred for the supplicants, she also opened the conversation between the gods and man. In the polis, ritual did not simply happen in the temple; the polis *was* the temple. In the sacred arena then, the priestess ensured the presence of divinity as the priest wielded the sacrificial knife. Rituals ensured every meal was blessed and offered in grateful thanks to gods and goddesses. As the priest plunged the blade deeply into the creature's flesh, the priestess released the death cry marking the transition of life to death.

Greeks never ate a domesticated animal without sacrificing it first and everyone in attendance at a festival was entitled to some portion of the meat. How big a cut of it, depended on their status. The highest citizens of the polis were given the entrails often to be used as omens by a priest or priestess called a haruspex. Bones were dedicated to the goddess and would also become a key tool for divination. The remainder of meat was shared between the worshippers, and as the flesh was consumed, so the people of Athens absorbed the elements of the gods.

Music, the Greeks believed, existed within any space where a deity and human met. It marked the space where the two communed. All music was deemed to be holy, and every ritual was accompanied by some kind of circle dance.

These cosmic dances sought to align humans with celestial planetary movements, dancing between each other in a predictable pattern so enormous, it became decidedly other. The universe was seen as circular. Every site was created with room for circular dances to take place in front of the altar, perhaps in memory of the dance floor that aids communication within the hive.

Imagine then, the scene. Melissae drum, setting the pace of conversation with the divine. Earth stands at the centre of the universe with planets rotating around her, protecting, nourishing, and caring for her inhabitants.

As Marija Gimbutas illustrated, everything in the ancient world worked towards a principle of cosmic wholeness. Ritual celebrated the sacred cycles of the Earth and then the arcane cycles of woman within that.

Ancient dance was a prayer. Graceful, eloquent, and full of humility. It communicated the collective reverence of the polis to The Goddess. How together they were grateful for her bounty, and as a unit, they longed for her grace.

Holding hands in circles, the dancers carefully choreographed movements mirroring the flow of energy around the world. Usually moving first to the right, suggestions have been made of an emulation of the route the sun takes across the sky each day.

According to sacred dance expert, Laura Shannon:

The concept of "right timing" was essential to ancient Greek ritual practices and remains important today. Ritual dance or any other ceremony still aims to bring about the experience of beauty and goodness which is summed up in the Greek word oraía (ωραία), from óra (ώρα), hour or season. The original meaning of oraía, "good", was "timely" or "ripe", occurring "at the proper moment" and therefore in the proper way.

Scholars propose certain dances may have been performed on specific dates, to align with each day's predominating constellations. Since festivals follow a moon-governed calendar, this seems plausible. And so, we imagine the Eleusinian initiates dancing around the well upon which Demeter was believed to have sat as she mourned her stolen daughter, with the lost child at the centre of her universe. Even today, it's still possible to see the wear and tear on the stones where hundreds of thousands of worshippers have danced around "The Well of Beautiful Dances".

But, of course, humans are not the only creatures who dance, and in fact the circle dance stands as one of the most important forms of communication in the hive. When a bee identifies a new pollen source, she takes a little taste of it back to the hive for her sisters. She has two dances to choose from to demonstrate where it came from, the figure of eight waggle dance, and for meals less than 500m from the hive, she uses a circle dance. First dancing right, in a circle, then back to the left, she tells the rest of the hive food is near and how to find it.

Chapter 8

Becoming an Ancient Greek Priestess

How women qualified for Athenian priestess roles varied. Certainly, families they were born into helped. Sometimes they inherited posts, presumably from their mothers, or occasionally lots were cast of applicants who qualified through ancestry.

Priesthoods could be purchased, and there is much evidence of that happening in the later Hellenistic era. When we consider the huge investments priestesses ploughed into cults, and that presumably cult and festival popularity could grow and wane, we can see how priesthoods could be massive drains on families' resources. Based on inscriptions, we know some families funded several cults at once.

Child

Between the ages of seven to ten, young girls were elected by a show of hands as to who would serve as *arrephoroi* – the carriers of the *arreta*, the "unnamed or secret things".

We know of two prominent functions of the arrephoroi.

First, they participated in the *Chalkeia*. Taking place in the months of *Pyanopsion* (end of October, beginning of November to us) the arrephoroi set up the warps (the threads going up and down) of the loom used to make a peplos, a robe worn by Greek women, to be sacrificed to Athena.

The peplos was woven into a representation of a battle of the giants called the *Gigantomachy*. During the skirmish between the Olympian gods and Gigantes, Athena was said to have launched her spear at Enceladus, disabling the offspring of Ouranos and Gaia.

Evidence suggests the arrephoroi, dressed in white, bestowed sacredness on the occasion, in the hope that The Three Graces might help the *ergastinai* – the women who were weaving – with their creation.

Every fourth year, the menfolk created a much larger version to sacrifice to The Goddess at the Panathenaea, a festival akin to the Olympic Games, which took place during subsequent months.

The other "main event" for the girls was the *Feast of the Arrephoroi* which took place at the end of the year (the night of the summer solstice), which seems to have been a nocturnal fertility rite symbolising human, animal, and vegetal increase.

In the days that preceded the festival, the girls were housed close to the temple on the Acropolis. Then during the feast, the priestess of Athena presented them with baskets containing objects (mysterious, even to her) for the arrephoroi to carry upon their heads out of the Acropolis. They would subsequently reappear through a vertical cleft in the rock that led them down to the gardens of the sanctuary of Eros and Aphrodite 300 yards to the east[34] returning with different baskets, again all covered up.

Suggestions as to what the arreta may have been, range from figures of snakes, young children, or male members, to live snakes or even a baby. A strange story, however, tells how the mythical associations of the Arrephoroi began with the three daughters of Kekrops, the first king of Athens, Aglauros, Herse, and Pandrosos. Athena had, just as the ritual demanded, given the girls their closed basket, which she had forbidden them to open. The temptation, however, had been too strong. Aglauros and Herse gave in to curiosity and sneaked a peek.

Inside, they saw Ericthonios, who had been birthed after Hephaestus had ejaculated onto Athena's leg one day. On wiping away the semen with a tissue, she dropped it onto the floor, and it had somehow impregnated Gaia. When snakes also appeared from the basket, the two girls jumped off the Acropolis to their deaths in terror. This myth is known as *Pandrosus* and within it Pandrosus means *"of the dew"* or *"all bedewed"*. Likewise, the daughters, collectively known as the *Kekropidai*, are sometimes called the "Dew Sisters".

It's likely that the legend may have had some roots in authenticity and that the arrephoroi might have originally been daughters of the royal family, which then got extended out to children of the priesthood or even handmaidens of the goddess. Virgins serving as arrephoroi were supported by liturgical fees. Both their own families and any other kin contributing toward their liturgies claimed her as a symbol of their wealth, and in turn as proof of their support of the polis. Ritual participants were highly valuable family resources; ones to be nurtured and protected. These girls were now set apart, different, and all eyes were now upon them.

As representatives of The Goddess, these girls would have brought great prosperity to their homes. Gold worn by the arrephoroi became sacred, and today we can still find seventeen of these girls by inscriptions on statue bases, set up by their families, in the Acropolis.

It's thought that after serving their terms as arrephoroi, the girls then progressed on to sacred grain grinders or *alteris*.

You might remember how, earlier, I spoke of a cup, depicting young girls running from the bear that seems to have depicted a ritual at Brauron?

At the sanctuary of Artemis Brauronia, girls from the ages of five to ten were cared for by a priestess who guided them through the awkward stages of childhood to puberty. Indeed, the myths tell of how, when asked by Zeus, what she would like from her life, Artemis asked to have 60 "daughters of *Okeanos*", all nine years of age, to be her choir.

The training of Lemon Balm tea's benefits for painful periods and mood swings would have been invaluable to these girls. I love to imagine it might have been given to them to drink.

Groups of youngsters were subdivided into ages to provide for a broader cult experience.

The very youngest served as hearth initiates at the Eleusinian Mysteries, offering prayers and sacrifices for the candidates, the *mystai*.

Interestingly, during Classical times, boys also tended the hearth, but by the Hellenistic period, all hearth initiates were girls. Families registered names of the children they wished to be considered for the post, and from them, one child would be selected by the Archon Basileus. Again, the children mostly seem to come from two clans: the Eumolpidai and Kerykes tribes.

By extension, we can see, too, how the young arrephoroi learnt the beginnings of a woman's trade, how to spin, to set up a loom, to weave and to grind the grain that would later be kneaded into bread.

Presumably, these girls weren't so different from kids today, being more willing to help somewhere else than tidying their own rooms at home. But when it came to helping with sewing and baking with their mothers, they had a deeper sense of sacredness in the work than we would have now.

Maiden

Now, a trap we can fall into in this work is to allow Romanising or Christianising attitudes to cloud our perceptions. This is particularly pertinent here.

One of the main ways priestesses have been undermined throughout history, has been by scholars trying to perceive their religion through the same eyes as we recognise our own. Until recently, most religious institutions excluded women from priesthoods, thus it was almost inconceivable it could have been any other way.

In fact, one of the first steps in eradicating the old religions to make way for the omnipotent male God was to eradicate priestesses, representatives of the image of the Great Mother.

In the Christian Church, chaste service to the Lord is a commitment nuns make for life. Conversely, chastity in the

Grecian priesthood was temporary and mostly only applied for the duration of a festival. Abstinence from sex was only expected for short periods of time, in most cases, for just a week before festivals commenced. Purification from relations was through washing and changing one's clothes. Sex was not seen as sullying, as opposed to something like a miscarriage was, for example: a "taint" seen as profound, and as such, requiring more help.

The Greek religion was fertile in essence, and as such, abundance did not only extend to the harvest but also the virility of husband and wife, and the happiness and productivity of the family unit. Lifelong priesthoods were typically held by married women who were otherwise going about their normal everyday lives.

In the few instances where continuous need for "virginity" would be required, such as to hold the position of the Pythia, the Oracle of Delphi, or the crone Melissa Chthonia, then older women were usually recruited.

Later, in Rome, girls as young as 6-10 took posts as Vestal Virgins which held a 30-year requirement of chastity, but no such obligation existed in the Grecian religion.

The ancient Greek *"Parthenos"* was simply a girl who had begun her periods but was not yet married. Unlike today, the term had no emphasis on her hymen needing to be intact.

Pausanias described that priestesses of all Artemisian cults were virgins, and that they held the post for a year. At Ephesus, these virgin priestesses were known as Melissonomoi.

Artemis was the guardian of young women, and at Ephesus, *parthenoi* are known to have been allowed to go on to marriage and motherhood after their year-long service, but the penalty for not remaining celibate whilst in the 12 months of service to Artemis was steep. Pausanias told the legend of one such priestess, Komaitho, from the ancient city of Patrai, modern-day Patras.

Melanippos and Komaitho had fallen in love, and Melanippos had sought Komaitho's father's permission to marry, but had been denied it. In rebellion, the star-crossed lovers began to meet in secret and have sex anyway inside the temenos, Artemis' sacred precinct.

The harvest caught a blight and began to fail, and when the people of Patras consulted Apollo's oracle, the couple's sordid behaviour was exposed and revealed as the root of the plague. To communicate their outrage at their beloved goddess' sanctuary having been so disgracefully violated, and to ensure it never happened again, it was decreed that the two should be sacrificed to appease her. Each year, thereafter, human sacrifices were offered as two youths were executed in penance of Komaitho's failings.

Pausanias, romantic old devil that he was, wrote:

The innocent youths and maidens who perished because of Melanippos and Komaitho suffered a piteous fate, as did also their relatives; but the pair, I hold, were exempt from suffering, for the one thing that is worth a man's life is to be successful in love.[35]

On rare occasions where "virgin priesthoods" do occur in mythology they carry different connotations. One example might be Herakles' impressive encounter with 49 of Thespius's daughters in just one night. The fiftieth girl didn't fancy it and stood her ground, rejecting him. Furious, he condemned her to service in his cult of Herakles Charops at Thespiai in Boitia, to serve the rest of her days as a virgin. Whether this priesthood truly existed outside of mythology, has so far not been discerned.

It helps to think of these young women as being of high school age. Different to our day, adolescence didn't exist. As soon as a girl started her periods, she was fertile enough to marry. The *parthenos* or maiden was at her prime, and a period of servitude gave her prestigious and beneficent options, to continue her priestess training, without the restraints of marriage, and thus to increase her power.

Festivals effectively functioned as platforms for the parthenos to showcase her skills. Disallowed from spending time unchaperoned, a maiden could demonstrate her culinary and craft abilities for any prospective suitor's family to purvey.

After all, if a maiden were to continue her career as priestess, a favourable marriage probably meant the difference between climbing to the most illustrious ranks or supporting another at the reins.

In his first century CE travel writings, Pausanias described several other parthenoi positions, all held for relatively short periods.

One such role was *plyntria*, sacred washer of the garments worn by Athena's statue. In Athens, this role commemorated Aglauros, the first priestess to have held the post. King Kekrops' daughter had attended to her duties well until, you may remember, she plunged to her death on the Acropolis. After her death, no-one thought to take over her duties, so the goddess' garments had gone neglected for a year. To ensure such a travesty could never take place again, an annual ceremonial washing of the vestments, *Plyntera*, was created. The festival spread and other Plyntera festivals are known of right across the Greek world. As *parthenoi plyntrides* washed the goddess' clothes, it was the job of another maiden, *loutrides*, to wash the statue itself.

At Didyma, in modern-day Turkey, the most prominent post for a maiden was *hydrophoros*, the water bearer for Artemis Pythia. An inscription found on the island of Patmos, just off the Turkish coast, tells us Artemis herself made Kydonia, daughter of Glaukies, into priestess and hydrophore. The queen who gave birth to her water bees.

The site of Lagina is an ancient Carian city, in Yatagan, in the province of Mugla. There, the most prominent maiden's role was *kleidophoros*, key-bearer. Interestingly this post was only available to the daughter of the priest of Hekate, meaning father and child worked together there.

At Sicyon, about 11 miles northwest of Corinth, a maiden could serve in a year-long office as *loutrophoros*, the bearer of the wedding bathwater for Aphrodite, under the supervision of a priestess of Demeter Kore, whose position as warden of the temple, was *neokoros*. Coincidentally, *Loutrophoros* is also the name of a kind of vase for carrying bathwater for a bride to bathe in before her nuptials.

At this stage of a young priestess' life, the most visible honour would be to be selected as *kanephoros*, or basket carrier. Almost every cult had a festival commencing with a procession where kanephoroi carried sacred objects from *here* to *there*.

In the case of Melissa serving at the Greater Mysteries, the procession followed the sacred way for fourteen miles from Athens to Eleusis, and her very presence at the front of the procession underlined the sacred connection the two cities had.

All eyes were on the priestess, as she heralded the beginning of the most impressive spectacle of the Athenian year. Glorious in her regalia, her face adorned prettily with white make-up, she encapsulated everything the Greeks felt was wondrous about their race.

These positions, *arrhephoroi*, *ergastinai*, and *kanephoros*, represented vital stages on the priestess' career ladder, and the polis bore witness to each rung she climbed.

To be chosen as kanephoros was the epitome of specialness. It set the parthenos apart as beautiful and select. Importantly, it also set them up as the most desirable of wives.

Sourvinou-Inwood begged us not to see through contemporary eyes, but it's irresistible not to compare our beautiful kanephoros with myself at that age. A member of the scouting movement, I was chosen several times to be standard bearer and to head up both the St George's and Remembrance

Sunday parades. A great honour, carrying the flag always made me extremely proud, but thinking about our Grecian maiden has encouraged me to try to extrapolate *why* it might have been me who was chosen.

Actually, thinking about it, I was also both May Queen and Mary in the infants' nativity too, which was no small feat when you think I'm not even from a Christian family. (Potentially my teachers came to regret that decision when I forgot the baby Jesus, so someone launched the swaddled doll from behind the scenes into the centre-stage manger and missed. But that's another story!)

Perhaps it was my looks. We might imagine that's what determined priestess selection too. My face has always been just the right side of plain and in those days, I curved in and out in the right places, but I can think of dozens of girls prettier than me.

But it wasn't *them* who were chosen to carry the flag. So why me?

My dad was scout leader, so I'd been part of the movement since I was born. Maybe that bought me some degree of nepotism from the decision makers, or I guess they recognised that might give the occasion more significance to me.

More likely, though, was all the drama, dance and singing classes I'd had throughout my childhood. I'd been groomed to be comfortable with all eyes on me, to pull my tummy in, lift my chin and walk with my head held tall. My posture was stronger, my presence brighter, and this stage brat didn't get distracted by crowds.

Were the young priestesses groomed to be stars?

I think so, potentially by strong mothers, themselves priestesses from prominent families, and indeed sources do attest that 80% of the parthenoi priestesses we know of today are proven to have been born from prominent families who also held other sacred offices.[36,37]

But if we're not careful, we fall into the trap of imagining all of this was just pageantry to secure themselves a man, but to quote Adam and The Ants:

Don't drink, don't smoke,
What do you do?
Subtle Innuendo follows
Must be something inside...

Left to their own devises, without the distractions of a man to care for or screams of marauding kids, the parthenos quietly practised womb shamanism, gradually learning control of her inner necktary and, in some cases, learning how to ravish nature with the lusty abandon of a bee.

Wife, mother

As we have seen, the highest-ranking priesthoods belonged to married women, especially in the cases of inherited offices, such as that of Athena Polis which relied on legitimate claim to the post through bloodline.

Married women played prominent roles in the cult of Demeter. The Goddess Of Fertility, Agriculture, and The Sacred Law had direct parallels with a woman's own cycles. The role of fertile, sexual women in the cult reflected the archetypal Mother Goddess herself.

The lifelong office of the priestess of Demeter Kore at Eleusis belonged to married women as did the roles of the two Hierophantide assisting her, and the priestess of Plouton.

They looked after the cult statues, decorating, and beautifying them.

Menopause

In some exceptional cases, certain cults required a commitment to chastity from a priestess which was expected to last longer than a few days. In these cases, older women were chosen, perhaps widows, who no longer felt the desire to have sex. Their moon blood replaced by "Wise Blood", in the eyes of the Athenians, they took on positions of great power.

We spoke of the Pythia being chosen from older women, as too were the priestesses of Demeter Chthonia. This office is remarkable because it's the only one we know of where the priestess actually carries out the ritual sacrifice of an animal, instead of a male priest.

Pausanias tells us that four chairs were set aside for the priestesses, who waited inside until the procession arrived. Worshippers led rowdy cows along the streets to the temple.

As the parade arrived, the doors were flung open, and the first cow was led in. Closing the doors behind them, Pausanias reports how the previously marauding cow suddenly went quiet and was led, serenely, by the ear to the altar, where it was slaughtered by these four crones. When the beast was finally dead, the doors were opened for the next creature to be led in.

Interestingly, in Paul Sédir's *Concise Guide to Medicinal Plants*, a 19th century CE work that merges botany with ancient, medieval, and Renaissance traditions of occult herbalism, he writes of the Lemon Balm plant:

> *This herb of rejuvenation was sacred to medieval magicians, who gave it the Chaldean name **celveios**. According to **Grand Albert**, wearing this herb as an amulet makes the wearer amiable and attaching it to the neck of an ox will follow you around wherever you go.*

(Grand Albert is a 13th century grimoire.)[38]

Could *Melissa officinalis* have been Melissa Chthonia's secret?

Chapter 9

Demeter and Persephone

Demeter's story is of a *vulnerable Goddess*. This title alludes to how her daughter was snatched away from her because of a heinous pact made between her father Zeus and his brother Hades. Many men had asked for the beautiful Kore's hand, but she had shunned them all. Hades was now determined, and since nobody was seemingly going to come up to Demeter's lofty standards, Zeus relented and agreed to give the hand of his daughter to the god of the underworld. Nevertheless, he knew getting the plan past Demeter was going to be a challenge.

One day, Kore, which means *"maiden"*, is walking with her friends in the Vale of Nysa, when she spies a narcissus, bends down, and plucks it. As she does so, the ground opens up, out roars Hades in his chariot who grabs and abducts her into the crevice, down into the underworld. In terror she screams for her mother, but Demeter doesn't hear her, and finally the Earth closes up and Kore is gone.

Poor Demeter cannot find her child. For nine days, she searches but nobody can help find Kore. On the tenth day, Hekate the goddess of witchcraft, reveals she heard the girl's screams from her cave as she stirred her cauldron, but did not see who took her. She suggests the sun god, Helios, might be able to help, as he sees all actions of gods and mortals in his journeys across the skies. And indeed, she's right; when asked, Helios tells how the girl was taken by Hades, but worse, with the consent of her father, Zeus.

Demeter is beside herself. Stripping away her goddess' garb, she dresses as an old woman, and searches and searches until she arrives at the town of Eleusis where eventually she finds a well where she can rest. Bereft, as she drinks, she sobs. Grief-stricken and full of rage she withdraws her fertility from the Earth and commits it to famine.

On fetching water for the palace, daughters of King Celeus discover the broken woman who is now calling herself Doso.[39]

The princesses are shocked at the awful tale of how this poor woman has lost her daughter. They head home to beg their parents to allow them to take her in.

On agreeing, the queen Metaneira cannot help but be moved by the desolate creature who stands, seemingly in a dream, before her. She offers her a chair, but Demeter refuses it. Unable to sit still, round, and round, she paces. Metaneira instructs her maid – Iambe – to fetch their guest a stool, which she does, and Iambe covers it in a soft white cushion of ram's fleece.

Metaneira offers her wine, but Demeter refuses it, explaining the only refreshment she desires is the kykeon – the Eleusinian barley drink. Iambe tries to cheer her, telling bawdy jokes and then eventually lifting her skirt to flash her genitals. Finally, the goddess laughs heartily, and her spirits start to lift.

Metaneira becomes impressed by this strange woman, so besotted by her child, and wanting to somehow distract her from her pain, Metaneira decides to place her in charge of her own child. She asks her to act as nanny to her son, Demophoon.

Yearning to repay the kindness of the woman who had sheltered her, Demeter agrees. Presumably wanting to protect her new friend from the horrors she had felt in losing her own child, she conspires to transform Demophoon's mortality into godliness. By night she places him in the ashes of the fire, gradually burning away his mortal essence.

One night, Metaneira walks by the fire and sees her son, lain like a log in the flames. Terrified she snatches him out, demanding that Demeter explain herself.

Incandescent with rage, Demeter removes her disguise, reveals herself as goddess and reviles their stupidity in insisting she make the boy mortal again. Now uncovered as a deity, she demands the king must instruct his people to build her a sanctuary. Therein she will reveal her secrets to them.

They do so, but poor Demeter simply sits in her temple and mourns, until Zeus finally realises that if the people starve, there will be no sacrifices so that will be the end of the gods too. Finally, he capitulates and sends Hermes down to the underworld to bring the Kore back.

Hades gets wind of the plan and has no intention of being duped, so gets her to eat four pomegranate seeds. (Some versions of the myth describe how some mischievous sprite may have done the tricking with his bidding and she may have eaten six – clearly the difference in seeds relates to how long you perceive that winter might be. Likewise, whether you feel she may have been tricked or decided to eat them of her own volition will inform your interpretation of who the Kore was at this point.)

An edict made by The Fates says that any food consumed in the underworld binds you to that place, so when she returns to the Earth, even though she is overjoyed, Demeter realises that Kore will, for ever, have to spend four months of the year, taking care of underworld souls in her elevated initiation as Queen of The Underworld, Persephone.

At this point, we should perhaps pause and contemplate the two obvious roles of the bee goddess. At the surface level, Demeter is an allegory for the insect's role in the harvest. Zeus used the same argument we still use today. If the bees are not kept happy, then food chains will inevitably suffer, but then he's wise enough to recognise the wider ramifications of the problem, that life as we know it will, to all intents and purposes, be over. More hidden, Persephone represents the bees' imagined role of psychopomp to the dead.

Returning to the myth, Demeter, appeased, returns her bounty to the Earth, allowing things to grow again. She then teaches Triptolemos – the father of agriculture (thought to be one of Metaneira's older sons who had been kindly towards her in her time of need) – how to farm the land and together they bring into life the first-ever grain crops, in the Rharian Fields.

Triptolemos, whose name means "He who pounds the husks", was provided with a winged serpent-drawn chariot so that he could spread the secret across all of mankind. At the start of his mission, he sowed the first Rharian Field, which was to become the sacred place of the Greeks. On his return to Eleusis, Demeter ordered King Celeus to surrender his country to him, in service for all he had done. In return, Triptolemos established worship to Demeter and instituted her sacred rituals of Thesmophoria.

The two best versions of the Demeter tale come from the second *Homeric Hymn* by Homer and Ovid's *Metamorphoses*, which is told with the Roman counterparts of Ceres and Proserpina.

Demeter is the archetypal mother Goddess. She was one of the 12 Olympian deities, Goddess Of The Harvest, Of Grains and of Fertility Of The Earth. This association with Earth meant she was important to peasant farmers. Ruler of plants, cycles, and seasons, she was seen as the protectress of crops. The grain fields and the threshing floor were her temple where she might manifest at any moment.

She had many names.

"Sito" – she of the grain, describing her as the goddess who feeds and makes things grow.

Sometimes "Green" and "The giver of gifts". Green is an interesting name because the colour is connected to the idea of things being *"other"*, indeed, belonging to the realm of The Fae. Sprites and faeries are often described as wearing green. The explanation of association with nature and growth is probably surplus to requirement here.

She is "Bearer of Food" and "Great Mother".

Surprisingly perhaps, considering her foul temper plunged the entire planet into famine, she is also referred to as "Good Mother".

She is "Thesmophoros" meaning divine order (Thesmos), "Legislator" and "Giver of customs". As Thesmophoros, she is law bringer, law bearer and keeper of the sacred laws. Thus, she is creatrix and mediator of civilized society.

The sacred laws were her purview, as was the realm of death.

She is a *chthonic* deity, meaning subterranean, but we can perceive it as meaning either "Earth" or more specifically "that which occurs *under* the Earth", or "as having a relationship with, or inhabiting, the underworld".

Chthonic deities tend to have been attributed a different kind of supernatural power, the awesome majesty of transformation. Interestingly, if we think about it from the perspective of analytical psychology, chthonic relates to our shadow side, that darker sense of nature within, not necessarily identified as bad nature, as opposed to good, but rather untamed, chaotic, and rampant.[40]

One of the six holy children, Demeter is daughter of Chronos and Rhea, born after Hestia and before Hera. Like the others, she had been swallowed and later regurgitated by Chronos, in his paranoia that one of his children would kill him, just as he had killed his own father, Ouranos. Later, thanks to Rhea's clever trickery, by inducing him to swallow a stone, Demeter was brought forth. Older counterpart to Dionysos, he and she are both gods of the Earth, and were worshipped together at the Mysteries of Eleusis. Importantly, like Dionysos' cult, Demeter's festivities were a group experience, hers with dry grain and his with the liquid of the grape.

When depicted, we usually find her fully clothed, wearing pretty, but matronly dresses, often wearing a wreath of corn. Sometimes she is seated alone upon her throne, others she is pictured accompanied by her daughter. She is occasionally also joined by Triptolemos who is seated in his chariot.

Her symbols are the torch and sceptre. The bee, pig and snake are sacred to her, as were barley, wheat, and poppies.

Karl Kerényi suggested that the Minoan poppy Goddess may have been transmitted from Crete and translated as the stories of Rhea and Demeter, to form part of the Eleusinian Mysteries. Poppies were offered as gifts to the dead and seemed to signify the blood of resurrection. According to Theocritus, Demeter was pictured bearing sheaves of wheat and poppies in each of her hands.

She had three main relationships, which brought forth children.

With the mortal Iasion, whom Zeus killed with a thunderbolt because he did not approve of the mixed race relationship. Already pregnant, Demeter gave birth to twins, Ploutos the god of wealth and Philomeus the god of ploughing.

She became the fourth wife of Zeus, with whom she bore Persephone.

Poseidon, her brother, pursued her whilst she was mourning the loss of Persephone. She changed herself into a mare, so he disguised himself as a stallion then raped her. Again, she became pregnant, this time with a nymph by the name of Despoena and a talking-horse called Arion.

Representations of Melissa

In the third century CE, Porphyry wrote:

The ancients gave the name of Melissae (bees) to the priestesses of Demeter who were initiates of the chthonian Goddess; the name Melitodes to Kore herself: the moon (Artemis) too, whose province it was to bring to the birth, they are called Melissa, because the moon being a bull and its ascension the bull, bees are begotten of bulls. And souls that pass to the earth are bull-begotten.

The association between Demeter and bees is undisputed. Her priestesses were referred to as Melissae, as was The Goddess, on some occasions too. Her daughter Persephone is known as Melitodes, literally *The Honeyed One*. Often, we hear of "Persephone's bees".

In Callimachus' Hymn to Apollo, we see the priestesses, or maybe actual bees, carry water to her:

And not of every water do the Melissae carry to Deo, but of the trickling stream that springs from a holy fountain, pure and undefiled, the very crown of waters.

Whether priestess or bee, we can draw associations between the liquids of this verse and water bees that bring fluids into the hive for the fanning bees that evaporate moisture from honey, into the air to eventually be rained sweetly back down onto crops and into rivers. Simultaneously priestesses who carry water for libations and rituals, and perhaps brides who will carry their bathwater to the Sanctuary of the Nymphs in offering to Artemis, the morning before their wedding. Perhaps too, we might consider how the Great Mother might appreciate the steady trickle of amniotic fluid. They are also *hydrophoroi*, the shapeshifting bee deamons, with tiny wasp-like waists, seen on many ancient Greek seals and stamps.[29]

In Servius's fourth century CE *Aeneid*, we discover Demeter initiated her original priestess, Melissa, herself and swore her to secrecy about the details of her initiation. Jealous and curious, the other women pleaded with Melissa to disclose to them what had happened to her, but she steadfastly refused to tell. Driven mad with frustration, the furious women tore her limb from limb. Demeter took vengeance by cursing bees to erupt from her severed head.

From Pindar's ode, *The Pythian*, we learn that women initiated into Demeter's mysteries, and especially her festival, Thesmophoria, are called bees, and so by extension the priestesses of the rite are also known by the name.

According to *The Homeric Hymn to Hermes*, and to Pausanias, Demeter's priestesses were the only women allowed to attend the rites of Dionysos, and in the days following The Eleusinian Mysteries, there was another exclusively women's festival, the Haloea, which celebrated Demeter and Dionysos jointly. That at least some of the benevolent Melissae may also have been the terrifying Maenads, who walked the shadows, seems likely, but it is not seen in literature.

Aspect of the Woman

Earlier, we focused on the priestess herself, what her duties were and some of the training she underwent to become that. But in this section, we meet the Melissa as your average, every day woman.

Melissa, lover of The Goddess.

When the High Priestess unlocked the temple doors and opened the sacred space, she sanctified an arena of privilege of speaking to Demeter. What sort of questions, concerns or even words of gratitude might our Melissa have brought before the goddess based upon the myth we just read?

She paid homage to herself as the matriarch, the loving mother, the jealous crone, the parts of her that were volatile and complicated and the unconditional love she has for her child. Likewise, her motherhood issues might have been in connection with her own mother and the stresses, strains and great opportunities that come from that relationship.

Perhaps the face of the goddess she saw reflected, might have been the propensity to be overprotective, oversensitive, or vengeful. Just as likely, there would be days when she recognised that she'd been enough; days when she'd been proud of her parenting or indeed of her children and wanted to give thanks for Demeter's help with that.

Fertility issues, of course, become part of that conversation; to want more children, to plead to the goddess to be overlooked and not to be given any more.

The sense of her own personal rhythms: her menstrual cycle, certainly, but unspoken conversations with the goddess also acknowledge the extrasensory nature of a woman as she bleeds and the changing landscape of her mind against the backdrop of the moon.

Externally, of course, fertility of their crops, and to have enough food to eat. To thank the goddess for the harvest, but in the winter to beg for her attention in the germination of the seed. To be present and generous in the weather to create exactly the kind of crop that they need. To protect it from pestilence, rodents, or insect and avian predation. To ask for her to intercede with the rain, to provide the sun, not too much though... just enough.

One might ponder, at this point, how exquisitely well ordered the honeycomb is. Any damage immediately being repaired. Thus, in honour and gratitude of Demeter's attention, and indeed in recognition of her propensity to manifest in the fields or upon the threshing floor at any time: the tidiness, the order, the care against fungi, moulds, rodents, and predators. The preparedness in the farming, in readiness for the Bee Goddess, as divine auditor, to appear.

And in the same way, we have seen the symbology becoming one... the grain goddess, woman, crops... so do the two become one. Ultimately Melissa and bee, working together, eventually transcending the one.

That the woman too, in her bleeding, acknowledges how much the goddess had done for her, stoops in the fields and returns her own life giving fluids back to the Earth. Replete with nutrients, blood, life, death, decay, and rebirth all become intertwined.

Always walking an infinite line between sacred and profane, our Melissa connects with her goddess, holds the divinity with her and brings it back into her everyday life, spinning it, drawing it, baking it, preserving it. When she rhythmically kneads her bread in her kitchen, the scent of the baking takes her thoughts back to the fertility of the goddess again.

The result of Demeter's union with Zeus was Persephone, also known by her childhood name Kore, or Kora. Later, she would morph from *The Maiden* to Queen of The Underworld, after being abducted by Hades, who took her as his wife.

Where Demeter is goddess of the harvest and fertility, Persephone is seen as the very personification of vegetation, returning from the underworld as the goddess of spring, inspiring plants to bloom forth and then, on the outbreath, reverting to her throne in the underworld in the dark winter months.

Like Demeter, Persephone is a chthonic goddess. In that sphere, she becomes a miraculous being, and thus, bringer of sorcery. It is in this guise that we should also view the Melissa High Priestess of Demeter Kore. As human proxy for the double goddess, she is seen as in control of motherhood and the harvest, and as being able to intercede with the god of the dead on their behalf. Bees, inhabitants of the underworld, were intimately connected with the despatch of old souls and bringing of the new. They were seen as psychopomps, just as Persephone was, and indeed the priestesses who stood in for her on earth. Here, the women performed the sacred act of soul midwifery communing with the souls of the dead and healing soul wounds drawn from this life and the matriarchal lineage.

Virgil described how bees acted as psychopomp for the soul, returning it to the place *"where there is no room for death, and where the souls fly free, ranging the deep heavens to join the stars' imperishable number."* Then when the time was right, returning some small filament, down from the heavens, unto Earth to one of those being born.

Persephone is usually depicted as holding a sheaf of corn; she is also sometimes illustrated holding a sceptre and small box.

Most famously Persephone is consort to Hades, Lord of the Underworld, but she has another lover who is spoken about less often, the god Adonis whom she and Aphrodite, the goddess of love and beauty, would be in a constant tussle over.

Adonis was Aphrodite's mortal lover.

Ovid's telling of the myth, from fifth century BCE, is that Adonis was born from a union between Myrrha and her father, King Cinyras. Some say Aphrodite's wrath had been inflamed because Myrrha had spurned her worship, others that Myrrha's mother, Cenchreis, had claimed Myrrha's beauty surpassed even that of the goddess. Either way, Aphrodite was none too pleased, thus she cursed Myrrha that she would, for ever after, lust after her own father.

Ovid opens the tale by warning the audience to prepare themselves because the story they are about to hear may horrify them. That a love between a father and his daughter is a beautiful thing, but Myrrha's crime is one of the greatest that could ever take place. What's more he refuses to place the blame with Cupid, whose arrow pierces Myrrha's heart, but instead tells the audience they should be angry at The Fates.

Many lines are contributed to Myrrha's to-ing and froing in anguish about her increasingly consuming love for her father until in the end, she has to confide in someone. She speaks to the family nanny about her anguish, who promises to keep her secret. Ovid describes how Cinyras even asked her, innocently, on one occasion, what kind of husband she would like, but still did not conceive of the depth of Myrrha's dark longing when she replied, "One just like you."

Continually, Myrrha tortures herself, until one day the nanny walks into a room to ask her a question, only to find her trying to hang herself. She recognises she has to do something for the girl she has loved and cared for since she was a child.

Eventually, the Ceres Festival came round. Ovid is a Roman writer. Ceres was the Roman personification of Demeter The

Goddess of Grain, so potentially the Cerealia may be what the Greeks knew as Thesmophoria. Ovid describes it as a seven-day festival where women should not copulate with their husbands, and instead take part in a nocturnal festival. Together they search for Proserpina, dressed in white, carrying torches. (It sounds the same.)

The nursemaid seizes the opportunity, and tells Cinyras that he need not go without, when his wife is away, since she knows of a young woman who has become infatuated with him, and if he would like, she could bring her to him under cover of darkness, but to protect them both, he must promise not to light a lamp. The identity of this woman must remain a secret.

King Cinyras is so blind drunk, he'll agree to anything, so Myrrha and her father copulate for nine (maybe 12) days in the darkness, until her father's curiosity gets the better of him, but his illumination is torturous. Poor Cinyras is horrified to discover who his bed partner has been and chases his daughter off with a sword.

Myrrha ran and ran, desperate to escape his wrath. Unbeknownst to her she had become pregnant with her father's child, and eventually, by the time she reached Arabia, poor Myrrha was heavy with child and could run no more. Falling to her knees, she pleads to the gods to help her. Their solution was to turn her into a myrrh tree, or some tellings of the myth say myrtle.

Either way, it was in that guise that she gave birth to a child, Adonis. Some versions of her story say that myrrh spice was the tears she cried during labour. How Adonis was born, again is the subject of contention. Ovid says a boar ran into the tree with its tusk, and to his surprise a baby pops out. Others say he was birthed by Lucina and the nymphs of childbirth. Regardless, it seems Adonis was left all alone in the world with a mother who was also a tree.

Meanwhile, one of Cupid's arrows had gone astray and this time it had grazed the heart of his mother Aphrodite. When she was walking one day, she discovered the babe and the hex of the arrow poured through her veins. She was so enchanted by the child that she had to take him. She put him into a chest and asked Persephone to take care of him and raise him.

But the boy was beautiful, the youth, magnificent, and the man, Adonis, became the stuff that could stir any creature's loins. And still he did because both goddesses became transfixed. Bitterly, they began to fight. Zeus interceded and decreed that Adonis would spend a third of the year with the goddess of spring, a third with the goddess of love, and the other four months he was free to spend with whomever he chose.

The divine agreement worked for a while. Adonis chooses to spend his remaining four months with Aphrodite, who was somewhat distracted by her love. She neglected her duties, so nobody ever saw her, preferring to spend all her time with Adonis, accompanying him on his hunts. But she was nervous of him taking part in such a dangerous pastime as this, and often used to plead with him to stop in case something awful should happen.

Then, of course, eventually, it did. One day Adonis was out hunting, and he was gored to death by a wild boar. There are differences of opinion as to where the boar came from. Some say it was jealously sent by another of Aphrodite's lovers, Ares. Some say it was Artemis who sent it taking revenge on Aphrodite for the death of Hippolytus, but finally suspicion falls on Persephone, who may have sent it to ensure that the underworld drew him back. We'll never know.

There are several historical variants of Persephone's name, including **Persephassa** (Περσεφάσσα) and **Persephatta** (Περσεφάττα). The Romans Latinised her name to **Proserpina** and aligned her with their Goddess Libera: Freedom.

Porphyry dubs her Melitodes – the honeyed one,[41] or *Despoina*, which means Mistress, or perhaps Mistress of the House.

Interestingly though, remember, Despoina was the daughter of Demeter and Poseidon (different parentage to Persephone). But it is as Despoina that Persephone is worshipped, alongside Demeter in the Eleusinian Mysteries. It was said that only those who were initiated would ever know her real name.

Pausanias discussed the conundrum. He explained that Kore had been born before Despoina but clarified that Kore and Persephone were one and the same. True to the vow of secrecy though, he does not reveal Despoina's true name.

According to one of the Orphic hymns, Persephone herself had a daughter Melinoe; some tales say she was the daughter of Hades, although some also interpret the father as being Zeus, as Zeus appeared to Persephone in the guise of Hades.

Persephone is related as having four children, Melinoe, Dionysos, Zagreus and Plutus.

Melinoe was The Goddess Of Ghosts And Spirits and was the ruler of *propitiation*, the offerings of appeasement made by a family for the souls of their dead.

Bees, as the embodiment of Persephone, become psychopomps travelling freely between the two worlds, guiding the souls of the newly dead, in response to the gifts given to the goddess.

We might also see her referred to as Melaina, the underworld aspect of Persephone, the part of us that brings nightmares and sends us mad.

Stories describe how dogs bark endlessly into the night as they perceive Melinoe wandering the streets, tailed by her entourage of ghosts; for her tribe are those unfortunates who are unable to rest. Those without proper funerals, those who plague the living because they have no recourse to find peace.

She appears in the Hymns to Orpheus. This translation of the hymn by University of California professor, Apostolos N. Athanassakis reveals the goddess to us.

I call upon Melinoe,
saffron-cloaked nymph of the earth,
whom revered Persephone bore
by the mouth of the Kokytos river

Karl Kerényi identifies Kore as probably being Mistress of the Labyrinth, who presided over the palace at Knossos in Minoan Crete. This, according to Hyginus, also identifies her with Ariadne. It was as Ariadne that she helped Theseus to hunt and defeat the minotaur, advising him how to find the labyrinth centre, then training him to use a silver thread to get out.

Kerényi describes an inscription at Knossos:

"To all the gods, honey ... [,] to the mistress of the labyrinth honey"; giving the Mistress equal respect to that given to the gods.

A statue found at Knossos is one of the earliest representations of the Bee Goddess/priestess we have, dating to around 1500 BCE.

Chapter 10

The Cult of Artemis

In *The Sacred Bee in Ancient Times and Folklore,* Hilda M. Ransome describes how the honey bee was understood to be the form that the human soul took when it descended from Artemis herself.

Archaeologist Marija Gimbutas contemplated Porphyry's writings by explaining:

> ... *we learn that Artemis is a bee, Melissa, and that both she and the bull belong to the moon. Hence both are connected with the idea of a periodic regeneration. We also learn that souls are bees, and that Melissa draws souls down to be born. The idea of a "life in death" in this singularly interesting concept is expressed by the belief that the life of the bull passed into that of the bees.*

Artemis was one of the most beloved deities of the ancient world. She was Goddess Of The Forest, Mountains, and Wilderness. Goddess Of Wild Animals, The Moon and Chastity, together with The Goddess Eileithyia, she was also Goddess Of Midwifery And Childbirth. Any deaths that occurred during pregnancy, or illnesses that befell women, were attributed to her.

She is always depicted as young, agile, and beautiful, usually in a forest setting. Her symbols were her bow and arrow, her quiver, hunting knives, deer, and cypress.

She has innumerable names, suggesting myriad attributes. So, it would be impossible to cover *all* her aspects in a book like this. We'll touch on just a few. Likewise, she was seen in a variety of ways at each of her different sanctuaries, thus there is a requirement to be quite stereotypical in the interpretations, which in itself presents its own challenges. At Arcadia for example, there have been more sanctuaries found dedicated to Artemis, than anywhere else. However, how they conceived of the goddess there, may not have been the same as she was worshipped at, say, Brauron, for example.

At Arcadia, she was worshipped as goddess of the nymphs. You might want to sit with that for a while. Considering all the Grecian meanings of nymph is quite informative here. Nymph might mean unmarried woman, nature spirit, unhatched bee. We will come to see that nymph also denotes an extremely accomplished priestess.

Most of Artemis' epithets allude to either the forest or some other aspect of the natural world, suggesting she was somehow seen as the awesome power of nature.

In total, it was said she had a train of 60 nymphs (all of whom were chaste) and she had begun to believe that she was given the role of midwife by the Fates after she helped her mother Leto to birth her brother Apollo.

Leto's pregnancy had begun before Zeus had married Hera, which riled Hera so much that she created problems right through Leto's pregnancy, forcing her out of Olympus and then cursing her that when she went into labour, she was forbidden to give birth on *terra firma*, which included any of the mainland, or any island at sea.

Poor Leto wandered the Earth, but no-one would take her in for fear of offending Hera. The vengeful goddess set up many sentries to prevent Leto from resting and even instructed the snake dragon, Python, to chase her away from Delphi. Eventually, worried for her, Zeus sent Boreas the North Wind, to carry her out to sea.

Finally, after drifting for hours, the goddess reached the desolate, rocky island of Delos. Having nothing to lose, being a floating isle, unattached to the ground, Delos allowed her in. Other goddesses began to gather, to help Leto in her hour of need, but Hera, determined to stay away, also managed to detain Eileithyia, the ancient goddess of childbirth. Leto first gave birth to Artemis, and then after another nine arduous days of labour, the young Artemis was able to help her mother to birth Apollo.

You might consider how drone bees, having far smaller mandibles, are unable to birth themselves, and thus need their sister workers to deliver them. To my mind that Artemis, who was a bee, birthed her brother is perhaps the most profound truth of the cultus.

Despite the safe delivery of her offspring, Leto's problems were far from over. Both her children became powerful archers to protect her honour. At just four days old, Apollo avenged his mother by killing Python, the serpent that had disallowed her from sheltering at Delphi. When Tityus, the Euboean Giant, tried to rape Leto, Artemis and Apollo retaliated, slaughtering him.

This violent pattern continued as the gods grew. Repeatedly, they were driven by murderous rages to protect Leto and defend her honour. One such costly jibe came from Niobe who boasted that she was more deserving of adulation then Leto, since she had birthed seven sons and seven daughters. The twins answered this by slaying all but one of Niobe's children, Apollo slew the males and Artemis the females. Perhaps this is where the tradition of attributing pregnancy-related deaths to Artemis derives from. Certainly, her arrows were thought to bring disease and sudden death to female babies and little girls. The idea that she had *sent* them, rather than perhaps was responsible for not foreseeing dangers ahead, might be pertinent here, since, unlike her brother, Artemis was never associated with anything oracular. (Apollo was said to have taken the place of Python after he slaughtered him, to issue oracles to the priestesses at Delphi.)

Artemis Ephesia

Artemis of Ephesos (or Ephesus to the Romans, now part of modern-day Turkey) is a notable example of Cybele being assimilated with an existing Greek Goddess. The Temple of Artemis would later become known as The Artemesium of Diana of the Ephesians, as referred to in the Acts of the Apostles. Diana would come to be the name Artemis would be called as part of the Roman pantheon, her temple, one of the Seven Wonders of The Ancient World.

Here, we see the moon Goddess, Artemis, honoured differently than in any other region or temple. What's more she was venerated in a space already dedicated as sacred to Cybele. The strange and enigmatic polymastoid (many breasted) goddess, Artemis of Ephesus.

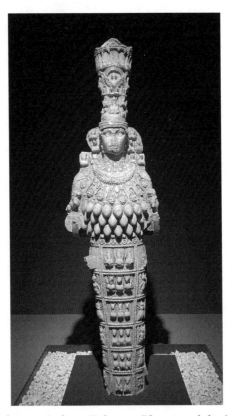

Statue of Artemis from Ephesus. Photograph by Metuboy.

To be clear, whilst Artemis was certainly worshipped differently here than she was in the rest of Greece, this is no offshoot fringe sect. The cult of Ephesus was colossal and bee motifs are everywhere.

The priestesses of Ephesus were called Melissonomoi (bees), and the chief priestess was referred to as The Beekeeper. Perhaps when bull worship was so strongly associated with Zeus, and bulls were believed to provide the origins of bees, it is not surprising that the priestesses of his daughter would come to be recognised as guardians of the souls of the underworld.[20]

At the new and full moons each month, the priesthood of Artemis conducted a night vigil and rites for her in the guise of "Queen Bee".[19]

Her priests were known as *Essene*, King Bee, the Greek word used to refer to drones.[29] According to Pausanias, their services were strict and puritanical. Just as Cybele had been before, the Ephesian Artemis was attended by eunuchs, this time known as Megabyzoi. It's interesting to contemplate that drone bees have no stinger either.

According to Autokrates, in *Tympanistai*, the priestesses in the Artemesium performed a waggle dance of their own, but not the usual figure of eight we imagine from the bee. He says:

As sweet maidens, daughters of Lydia, sport and lightly leap and clap their hands in the temple of Artemis the Fair at Ephesus, now sinking down upon their haunches and again springing up, like the hopping wagtail.[19]

If we leave the history and go back to entomology for a moment, there is a clear allegory that Artemis, who liked to go off and hunt alone, might be seen as another kind of insect.

Solitary Bees total roughly 250 of the bee species and can be divided into three classes: Leaf-cutters, Miners, and Masons.

As guardian of the medicinal plant knowledge, Artemis is most assuredly the leaf-cutter bee, held in great reverence by the people of Ephesus whose city and temple's architecture and superlative stone workmanship paid homage to the rest of the allegory... the Miners and the Masons.

Perhaps one morning, when dew sparkles like diamonds on the green carpet, you might hear a bee hum. Not nestled between the petals or snoozing, holding another bee's feet, but gently, carving out tiny images of her own goddess to take home.

Maybe you might even bend to look closer and whisper hello, but then notice your visitor is not who you thought. For your artistic friend, carefully sculpting tiny images of the moon in the leaves of your rose, isn't Apis mellifera, she's a leaf-cutter bee, a solitary bee who hunts for plants to build beautiful organic temples and prefers to live alone.

Leaf-Cutter Bees

Leaf-cutter bees belong to the Megachilidae family, and as solitary bees, do not live (like honey bees do) in social collectives. Most prefer to move into existing abandoned colonies, to live alone simply caring for their offspring. The Megachilidae family is a cosmopolitan lot with members from all over the globe. Different from other species, they collect pollen on their abdomen on a brush-like mechanism called the scopa.

The hairs on the scopa (plural scopae) are electrostatic. They have a top layer of long, stiff hairs to grab onto the pollen and floral oils are then absorbed into an underlayer of short, flexible hairs. The bottom layer can be made up of separate hairs or hairs branching off the upper layer. Scopa studies are an extraordinary thing in their own right, demonstrating just how wondrous evolution is. Species of bees that collect small pollen granules have denser, multibranched scopal hairs in comparison to those that have evolved to forage for larger grains. So, where bumblebees and honeys collect pollen into baskets on the backs of their hind legs, then tamp it down with drops of nectar, leaf-cutters wriggle it all onto their "tummies".

With some notable exceptions like Coast Leaf Cutters for example, who will make their nests in groups, most female leaf-cutters live solitary lives, tending their nests alone.

It seems to be a universal thing that bees like to go where bees have been before. We see it in honey bees who will happily move into a log that other bees vacate, and leaf-cutters are just the same. They like to discover a place where a colony has been before, move in, re-excavate, and then build their own lovely cells.

Dead wood, hollow plant stems, in the soil and sometimes in little cavities in walls all make lovely places to build a new home. Please think of the leaf-cutters when cutting dead stems in spring. The chances are you may have a number of friends who are hiding out.

The most common species in the UK is the delightfully named **Patchwork Leaf-Cutter**, who could be quite easily mistaken for a honey bee since they look so alike but she has two rather adorable qualities that may help you to recognise her if you take time to sit quietly and watch.

The first is she has a rather unusual feeding position. As she sups nectar, she lifts her abdomen up and down. She almost looks as if she is wagging her tail as she forages.

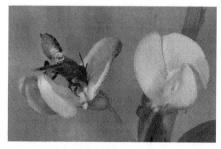

Leaf-cutter bee with pollen on her scopa. Photograph by Vijay Cavale.

Watch long enough and you might even witness her clipping delicate pieces from your roses and shrubs, then carrying them underneath her body to stash them in her nest. When back in her home, she makes a gossamer fabric, carefully gluing all the pieces together to construct cells into which she lays her eggs. She then fills the cots with pollen to ensure her offspring will have plenty to eat when they hatch. Deftly, she overlays each leaf with another and creates a kind of cigar shape. Amazingly she arranges the leaves just as if she is making a new rosebud, lays her egg, then places the final piece into it, to close the end. She will likely lay 20-30 eggs in each nest.

We have focused on Artemis the huntress, but she has another title too, more related to her function in relation to The Fates. As Artemis-Diana Eulinos/Eulinon, whose name translates as "She, the clever spinner", she also brings to mind another insect – The Wool Carder Bee, again a member of the Megachilidae family. This lovely girl, often seen in our gardens with a ginger bum, strips hairs of plants like lamb's ears, to cushion her luxurious nest. This one doesn't have a scopa and relies on energetically "swimming" in the flower to harvest its pollen.

Mason Bees

"Mason bee" is the common name for the species, *Osmia*. The genera, which comprises around 300 species in the Northern Hemisphere, is commonly called Mason because this bee likes to line the insides of her nest with mud.

Osmia means smell and relates to the aroma of the Nasonov she leaves at the end of her nest so she can always identify it when she returns from foraging. (That's a real Melissa loop, isn't it?!) Studies show that if a gardener happens to move her bamboo canes around, she can still locate and return to her own.

She lays one egg into each cell, which will hatch and pupate over the colder months, and then emerge in the spring. She cleverly lays females at the back of the nest, working towards males at the front. The males emerge first, wait for the females to appear, then hastily mate.

Shortly after mating, the drone dies. So, to all intents and purposes, she spends her whole existence living and working alone. Her industry is hard, making many journeys back and forth to gather enough pollen to fill each egg.

Over the year, she will potentially create around ten nests, capping each one before moving on to the next. Osmia are very unlikely to sting you. They are docile and friendly bees.

Miner Bees

Andrena, better known as mining bees, belong to the largest genus in the family *Andrenidae*. Found in most regions of the world with the notable exceptions of South America and Oceania, *Andrenidae* is one of the largest of all bee genera, comprising of over 1300 species.

Most commonly, Miner bee species will be brown to black in colour, but can be reddish, or sometimes even green or metallic blue. In all cases they will have a whitish hair band that stretches across their abdomens.

Miner bees have scopal hairs on their hind legs and hairy faces. They have a kind of mono brow that skirts round their eyes and under their antennae.

They like sandy soil to build their nests into, and you'll most likely find these near to or under shrubs, to shelter them from the frost and heat. After digging each cell, they fill it with pollen and nectar, lay an egg and then reseal it.

Similar to other solitary bees, they emerge in the spring, mate and lay eggs which pupate, and the next generation emerges the following spring.

A recent fascinating discovery is that, sensibly, in my opinion, Andrena mostly desire rose pollens. More recently though, as summer moves on, they become better behaved and start to collect more Brassicae family. Scientists suggest the species may have evolved to take advantage of the plentiful supply of oil seed rape. (*Brassica napus* subsp. *Oleifera*.)

Solitary bees have slower life cycles than their honey bee cousins. Each egg laid during the summer, hatches, and gorges itself, then pupates through the autumn and winter to emerge as a bee the following spring. Just like the parthenos priestess' service to Artemis, the life cycle of a solitary bee is a year.

Leaf-cutters are incredibly busy bees. Research shows just one will carry out the same amount of pollination as 20 honey bees. Their favourite haunts for pollen are on runner beans and other legumes, bramble blossoms and berry flowers. Attract solitary bees to your garden and they'll reward you by pollinating many species of fruit, vegetables, and wildflowers.

What delicious bounty from the goddess that is!

Insect bliss over, let's head back to Ephesus.

Some scholars suggest the many breasts on the statue may perhaps show where bees had originally built nests onto one of the older cult figures destroyed by the Cimmerians. Wild bees, regarded as holy, make egg-shaped nests. They are notorious for being ferocious when angry. Other suggestions offered up have been that they may depict bulls' testicles, grapes, or gourds, all which have long associations with the tradition. I think whichever you decide, they all come back to the same place, the idea of fertility.

That original statue was carved from wood, by a sculptor known as Endoeus, who had been a student of Daedalus. The likeness of The Goddess was adorned with jewellery made of all manner of precious metals. When the resting place of the statue was found during excavations, the carved idol had rotted away but its treasury of accoutrements remained just as they had been, when the priesthood had carefully dressed and hidden her for protection two millennia before.

In later incarnations of her likeness, ferocious beasts and bees adorned her skirt. The frame of her stature seems to echo the shape of a sarcophagus, and in some of her statues she wears a round temple or a tower upon her head.

Above her breast she wears a zodiac, symbolising *Logos*, the principal teaching of her sanctuary. Its beautiful wisdom displayed for all to see on her garb. How much of the zodiac is shown on statues differs, but invariably, sitting mid, front and centre is the sign of Cancer.

In total, around 600 of these bizarre-looking statues have been found around Greece attesting to the spread of her cult. Pausanias described how he knew of images of Artemis Ephesia in the government offices of Megalopolis, in the marketplace in Corinthos and in a village in Arcadia called Alea.

Her rituals weren't open to everyone. The cult of the Ephesian Artemis was for young women only. It was said that only unmarried women were allowed to attend, so amongst other ritual activities, it may have been here that they learned the secrets of Lemon Balm, the moon and menstruation.

It's also been suggested that some of the festivities may have included an opportunity for young women to meet their fiancés, an attractive aspect that probably helped to drive the popularity of the cult. Supposedly some gatherings were attended by the Kouretes, the mythic sons of Rhea, not priests, but rather young males who also offered sacrifices to the goddess.[42]

According to Dr. James Rietveld in *Artemis of the Ephesians*, the kouretes "inspected sacrificial victims, heralded the sacred at the Mysteries, were in charge of burning incense while a cultic dance was performed, played the flute as the libations were poured, and, most importantly, initiated people into the Mysteries."

Incredibly, even shields used by the Hoplites (warriors) of Ephesos displayed the bee motif, which might also suggest that Artemis retained Cybele's warrior dimension. That idea would also seem to be echoed by the fact she is clothed with and surrounded by ferocious, wild beasts.

In his 1939 paper, "The Bee of Artemis", G.W. Elderkin proved that linguistically, the name Ephesos translates to *"the place of many bees"*. He dissected some inscriptions to Artemis and found linguistics suggesting the older Lydian name may actually mean "Keeper of the Hive" and would relate to the goddess and her priestesses.

The Beekeeper Priestess

The yearlong service of chastity of a priestess of Artemis matches to the life cycle of a solitary bee. The *parthenos* is yet to be married and have a family of her own. To be clear though, the term is chaste, not virgin. There is no written requirement for the hymen to be intact, merely celibate for the year.

The leaf-cutter bee cuts half-moons, and Artemis is connected to aspects of the moon. Specifically, her day was the sixth of the month (remember the month starts at new moon). The shape of her "waxing" crescent is a close correlation to the moon-shaped leaf she cuts.

A human pregnancy is 40 weeks, ten moons. (Makes more sense than our 21st century counting towards labour, doesn't it?)

If the women communally bled at the dark of the moon (ritually or otherwise), the full moon would be their most fertile time. Thus, it seems likely that the period of confinement, would be expected to end at the full moon. Artemis' day is the 6th of the month because it was said she was born on this day. If babies were usually expected at the full moon, the 6th day would be an excellent marker for preparations. (Providing baby had read the textbooks, of course.)

That the bee creates a moon-shaped layette for her young is beautiful and really informs the way children were seen in Greece. At Thesmophoria, the priestesses also made their own beds from lygos leaves, perhaps in recognition of their place as daughters of the bee goddess.

Usage of lygos *(Vitex agnus castus)* to bring women's menstrual cycles into alignment is attested to by Theophrastus and Pliny, but any actual treatment must surely have taken place, privately, at home, rather than as part of the ritual, since sitting on dry leaves on the grass will have little or no effect on hormonal balance. Nevertheless, their cycles were believed to be in line with the moon and the lygos tree could have supported that happening.

If that were so, then they ovulated communally, at any ritual which may have taken place in the run-up to the full moon. All of female Athens was collected together at the height of their fertility to use it, not for sex, but for *impersonal* sex. Using specific meditations, visualisations and sheer willpower, they poured their collective sexual energy back into the Earth at the time it needed it most, just before the sowing. Instead of using their precious opportunities to make children, each woman gifted her most sacred monthly treasure to their Great Mother, as their personal contributions to provide for the polis through the year.

Just as Artemis was intended to be as wild and free as the uncultivated realms beyond civilization, so the parthenos owned her sovereignty.

That first sign of menstrual blood signified that maidens were ripe for wedlock[19] but Pliny the Elder described their belief that menstrual blood had magical properties and was responsible for increasing agricultural success. Moreover, women's fluids were even thought to influence the weather. He states: *"Over and above all this there is no limit to woman's power,"* for *"they say that hailstorms and whirlwinds are driven away if menstrual fluid is exposed to the very flashes of lightning; that stormy weather too is thus kept away, and that at sea exposure, even without menstruation, prevents storms."*

The sheer power of energy that floods down to the vagina, in some of the meditations, is every bit as blissful as sex. A woman entirely in control of her sexuality as sovereign. No wonder men would eventually feel the need to put an end to that.

Pleiades

In the myths, Artemis has a close relationship with the Pleiades, and oddly, Aristotle also seems to associate them with the return of the bees in spring. In *History of Animals*, he describes how there will be no honey in the hive until the Pleiades rise, then also Pliny depicts the constellation as a cluster of golden bees.[24]

Aristotle seems to have been besotted by bees. He was utterly fascinated by their quandary. In *Metaphysics* he debates for pages upon pages about how a species needs two sexes to reproduce, male and female, but bees, he insists, have three – King, worker, and drone. He hypothesises about all the ways they might mate, but he can't quite make it stick. He muses on many suggestions he's heard; like Virgil he speculates that perhaps bees might be deposited onto leaves fully formed. This of course is in opposition to Pliny who described the chrysalis stage of the bee.

Hesiod states that the Pleiades set in November, just around the time of Thesmophoria. Every constellation enjoys a period of invisibility in the sky. For the Pleiades that period lasts about 40 days.[43] Axial precession of the equinoxes affects when this invisibility will take place. This precession refers to the gradual shift in the orientation of Earth's axis of rotation within a cycle of approximately 26,000 years.

In the era of 3300 BCE, the heliacal rising of the Pleiades – when they can be seen at the horizon just before dawn – took place at the Vernal Equinox; its annual reappearance marked the return of spring. Aristotle seems to have been right. The Pleiades do seem to have brought the bees.

My choice of the date 3300 BCE was not arbitrary. I took it from a paper by T.D. Worthen, classics scholar from The University of

Arizona. In it, he attempts to establish an astronomical key to tie the dates of the Pleiades and the Hesperides. Presumably, like me, he too was irked that Virgil's information in the *Georgics*, about what to farm when, no longer matched, since the reason for this is this axis of precession.

He chose this era as the anchor point for his work because it corresponds to the diaspora of the Indo-European ancestors of the Greeks.

What's incredibly strange... nay, what's utterly bizarre, is... We can trace the name Pleiades to, and I quote...

a pre-Greek etymon which means "first" and connects it to an early Persian asterism (a cluster of stars that's not a constellation) by the name of *Purviyoni* which means "first vagina".[43]

It gets stranger.

In mythology, the Pleiades or the Seven Sisters are these nymphs who are Artemis' playmates along with their sister nymphs the Hyades – the rainmakers.

The Seven Sisters are Maia (Grandmother), Alcyone (Queen who wards off evil), Electra (Flowing), Asterope (Twinkling), Taygeta (Long-necked), Celaeno (Swarthy) and Merope (Bee-Eater).

Their father was Atlas, The World Pole, The Axis Mundi.

Merope

Merope – or *Bee Eater* – is the palest of the stars in the Pleiades. Merope had been associated with the bee-eater in the ancient Minoan language, long before the Hellenes had arrived.[44]

She gained her name as the "Lost Star", because astronomers didn't initially chart her with her sisters. She is imagined as spinning away from the rest of her family in shame since each of the other nymphs had given birth to children fathered by the gods, and Merope was said to have married a mortal.

Merope is the spinning star.

Her name is interesting. It means "honey faced", so we wonder if it might be related in the same way as the classicists related it to poetry and music? For example, how the bees kissed the lips of the muses. I wonder too if this might be an allusion to some kind of bee-mask used for shamanistic mummery.

That the giant, Orion, chases the Pleiades might also be engaging. Mythology places Orion's birthplace on Hyria in Boeotia. Homer talks about Hyria, when he lists the ships that were sent out to bring the beauteous Helen from Troy. Hesychius tells us that the related word *Hyron* is a Cretan word which can mean one of two things, either a swarm of bees or beehive.[44]

Now, the source I got this thread from, asks something very clever. It says:

Surely Merope the bee eater is unlikely to always be a bee herself. There is a small Mediterranean bird called the Bee-Eater, which was known under that name to Roman naturalists Pliny and Aelian, this Bee-Eater is most likely to have been a She-Bear, a representative of Artemis.[45]

I stared at this for hours because I couldn't see how the author had made that leap, but they are right... Artemis is a bee and a bear. We know all about the Brauronia festival, don't we? The girls running from the bear etc...

It must be right.

Merope must surely be Artemis.

Now, one thing I have come to know is the same truths are often echoed in other shamanistic oral traditions. Sometimes if you visit other nations' myths then, they might cast more light.

Here is a fitting example. The Kiowa tribe are indigenous peoples of the Great Plains of the United States. They migrated south from western Montana into the Colorado Rocky

Mountains in the 17th and 18th centuries. Finally, they reached the Southern Plains by the early 19th century.

They have a story about how the Pleiades had been placed in the sky when winter had come, one year, and their ancestors felt they should keep moving south for safety. Eventually they found a place that felt right to settle, so they made camp, but the place was already inhabited by bears.

By and by, they settled, but then one day, seven little girls were playing by the stream when bears emerged from the woods and chased them. The terrified girls leapt onto a rock and begged Great Spirit to protect them.

Great Spirit, on hearing their cries, decided the best way to help the girls would be to put them out of reach, so made the rock grow up and up, until its vast sides were almost vertical. As it grew, the girls were raised up out of the bears' reach.[46]

But the beasts were tenacious, clawing and scratching at the rock. They left deep scratch marks, but the rock just kept getting taller, pushing the seven little girls right up into the stars.[46]

That reminds me of the description of the young girls' ritual at Brauron, and as such, it would explain why they jumped on the rock. I'll add to that, in a moment, with some archeo-astronomical evidence from Artemis' shrine at Ortega.

"The Honey Bear" website tells how, in later times, there would be a recommendation written into a Syriac Book of Medicine that you should place a bear's eye into a hive to ensure that bees prosper. It says:

> *The bear's spirit apparently watches over the hive and this was precisely the Merope's role among the Hyria at Chios.*

Let's summarise and see if the clues do add up.

Does a bear have a honeyed face? It absolutely does. It smashes logs apart shovelling in the honey complete with bees, so that means it's also a bee-eater.

So that works.

But how does that equate to it protecting the hive?

We need to think like beekeepers (remember Artemis *is* the Beekeeper) and consider some aspects in terms of apiary hygiene.

Hive frames should be changed every couple of years, otherwise it leaves it open to infection and invasion from pests. One of these pests is called a **Wax Moth**.

The moths would be useful in the wild, after the bear had visited, since it feasts on wax, and thus it tidies up after the bees. In the hive though, it is a terrible nuisance, leaving silk trails all over the comb which eventually sabotages the health of the colony. An indicator moths are in residence is they gouge out claw-like marks all over the wood of the hive.

Wax moths particularly like places where brood have been raised and seek out comb that has had pollen within, in the past. They lay their young close to where bees are so their young can predate on honey bee larvae. (Remember, the bear ritual at Brauron was done annually by little girls.)

The moths lay their eggs into cracks that bees can't get into. When the eggs hatch, the moth larvae burrows through the brood comb almost as if they have woven across it. They feast on beeswax and honey bee cocoons left over from larval metamorphosis into bees. In some ways they are useful because their larvae consume bee faeces and cocoon silk, but in doing so they release these sticky trails that the bees struggle to clean off the comb.

Worse, the sticky substance traps adult bees inside their cells, meaning they die in them. These adult bees are later removed by worker bees. but it has the general effect of lowering the bee population and compromising colony health, making it more vulnerable to parasites, pests, and predators.

Moths seem to prefer dry combs to wet ones, and always prefer brood comb to honeycomb. The best way to check no larvae are hiding in nooks of the combs, if using from year to year, is to freeze them. Interestingly, that is reminiscent of a ritual custom of the priestesses at Brauron. They symbolically shrugged off their saffron robes to stand naked into the cold, in allegiance to Iphigenia, a priestess whose life Artemis once demanded after being betrayed by her father Agamemnon. She was grabbed by sentries and tried to escape by slipping out of her robes. Whether that's coincidence is hard to say, but it does seem to me to be reminiscent of removing the silk that may have trapped a fellow sister bee.

So, Aristotle said that bees seem to arrive with the heliacal rising of the Pleiades which are found in the constellation of Taurus. Bees which bring the souls are born from the carcasses of bulls (Taurus?).

Does that mean that's where the Greeks believed souls to come from too?

Nope.

Platonists believed the highest point of heaven, the gateway through which souls descended, was a constellation called Praesepe. Older than the Pleiades at an age of around 790 million years, Praesepe (which is Latin for "Cradle", or "Manger" derived from *Phatne* – from the Greek word to eat – *pateomai*) is a cluster of 1000 stars in the constellation of Cancer, located about 550 light-years from Earth. This cluster, of which 40 stars can be clearly seen with the naked eye, appears as a little patch of bright haziness during July and August. It was first identified as a group of stars by Galileo, but it was already included in the earliest known star catalogue written by Hipparchus in c. 129 BCE.

Found in the seasonal sign of Leo and located in the constellation of the Crab (Cancer), Praesepe is easy to find. First find the twin stars Castor and Pollux, then look to the east to locate Regulus. Cancer itself is not a bright constellation. The womblike darkness of the feminine sign has very few stars, so when the moodiness of astrology melts with dark astronomical skies, it really does translate into being a foreboding sign.

Praesepe pops prettily in the darkness.

Pliny writes:

If Praesaepe is not visible in a clear sky it is a presage of a violent storm.

The constellation is known today by the catalogue numbers NGC 2632 and M 44.

It does have a more common name.

The Beehive.

I kid you not. *The Beehive!*

New souls are brought down by the bees, from a place in the sky that is called the beehive. The beehive is in Cancer that stands at the centre of Artemis Ephesia's zodiac neckpiece.

So, I keep thinking – if they come from the beehive, where do we go to when we die?

Well, according to the Platonists, departing souls ascend back through the highest point of the heavens – through the Gate of The Gods – to the place they knew as *Capricornus* or Capricorn.

In through Cancer, the astrological mother, out through her opposite sign Capricorn, to the care of Hades, the god of the Dead, who would come to be Christianised as Satan, personified as a goat, the sigil of Capricorn.

Salutaris

Perhaps the greatest of all Artemisian rituals was the Salutaris procession. An enormous affair, effigies of Artemis and other supporting dignitaries were paraded throughout the city. It was quite the Grecian Hall of Fame, 29 statues of their illustrious and finest characters from mythology as well as past Emperors and members of their senate.

Austrian archaeologist Anton Bammer described in *Ephesos* that processions that led up to the great Altar of Artemis followed a set structure. Parthenos led, carrying baskets containing incenses and sacrificial tools, including knives and axes, and other unnamed tranklements. Musicians followed, then sacrificial animals dressed in garlands were led up accompanied by the sacrificial officer, usually a priest. Behind them, were flute-players who would play during the slaughter, then finally came the participant citizens.

A real *Star-Spangled Banner* moment. *Land of Hope and Glory*. A strong and resilient hive.

The statues of Artemis gradually increased in splendour, presumably in testament to the strength of the nation, gradually becoming increasingly more elaborate. Beginning with statues of wood and stone, through to silver, the opulence of the procession climaxed with a triumphant golden statue of Artemis the Huntress, complete with her burning glow.

Sparking the dying rays of the evening sun, it must have looked breathtaking.

The procession was led by the *dadouchos* (torch bearer) wielding a flaming torch which could hardly be seen in the early moments, gaining brilliance as the skies turned inky behind it.

The route began as united – then split at Mount Pion with one route looping south to the Corresian Gate and the other heading north to the Magnesian Gate then circling round towards Mount Pion.

The territory around Magnesia was lush and fertile, producing fabulous cucumbers, wine, and figs. Built downstream from Ephesus, on the banks of the tributary of the Meander River, on the slope of Mount Thorax, it sits just 15 miles from the honey sounding city of Miletus. I can find no geographical reference to anywhere called Mount Thorax, but strangely it is the anatomical part of a bee. Bees have heads, bodies, and thoraxes.

Six gorgeous Greek statues were unearthed in the ruins of Artemis at Magnesia of the Meander. The discovery is very reminiscent of Aristotle's musings about the sexuality of the hive. Four of the statues were female, one was male but the gender of the sixth one could not be determined.[47]

However, Magnesia… that horrid medicine taken for heartburn and constipation, milk of magnesia… chalky, right? Vile…

I wanted to find out whether the spectacular gate they had processed through was made of limestone, and yes, it was. Apparently, over the centuries, it had suffered quite a bashing from thieves and lime burners. I'm not sure whether there was a quarry nearby or not, but strangely, Magnesian limescale came from England – Yorkshire.

Limestone is chalk.

That makes me think of a fungal infection that kills bee larvae called *Chalk Brood*.

Young, infected larvae usually show few symptoms of having any kind of disease but then, to all intents and purposes, they kind of suffocate in their combs. Because they cannot moult their pupae, they effectively get sealed within their tombs. The tops of the cells go all sticky, sort of fall inwards, and look like the rind of Camembert cheese.

What do you think the undertaker bees find when they uncap dead larvae cells?

I'll give you a clue. If this were the cult of Osiris and there was a tomb, what would you expect to find? One can but marvel at the similarity between the metamorphosis of bee larvae and bodies wrapped in bandages.

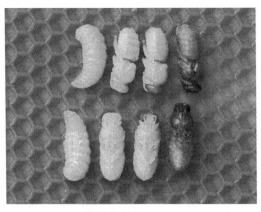

Metamorphosis of drone larvae. Photograph by Waugsberg.

The remains of the bees that succumbed to this disease look like, and are called, mummies.

Since bees are such good housekeepers, they won't tolerate these in the hive, so they chuck them out. Tiny pieces of chalk accumulate on the ground all around the hive.

So, what can you do about chalk brood? Well...

Whilst it doesn't kill the colony, it does weaken it, and one of the best preventions is to ensure you have a strong robust colony. Maybe a round of *Land of Hope and Glory* would do it, and you should always burn infected frames. That'll be another association with the torch then!

Finally, most people agree that you shouldn't raise a queen from chalk brood. Commercial beekeepers would say it was better to requeen; bee guardians would trust that the worker bees will be able to raise a new princess capable of taking the place, or at least supporting the dowager.

Hence:

New Artemis.

New Artemis.

New Artemis, until you have the best queen you can get.

Likewise, if several virgin princesses hatch, only the strongest and most capable can survive. She is the golden queen.

Beekeepers, though, here's a question for you.

If, and I stress *if*, what we're seeing here is chalk brood, what are you going to do about it? You've cleaned, burned the frames and you've requeened.

You want a prevention, yes?

Some keepers suggest using essential oil constituents.

Thymol. (Found in thyme. Also fabulous against parasitic varroa mites and box caterpillars, I hear.)

Given that, what do you think the city of Ephesus are famous for selling?

Ephesian honey tastes of thyme.

What do you think? Have I produced a decent argument?

I'm quite happy with it, I've got to be honest, but there is a problem.

Presumably the disease existed before the fungus causing chalk brood *(Ascophaera apis)* was identified in 1913; nevertheless, it would be difficult to prove exactly how far back in time people were noticing the first bee mummies.

Chapter 11

Divination and Oracles

In *Ancient Greek Divination*, Sarah Iles Johnston conveys divination's position at the very centre of the Greek religion. She speaks of four key oracular centres at Delphi, Dodona, Claros and Didyma, and states a case for institutional oracles and freelance diviners. This is interesting because it gives us a new slant on this idea of so many Melissae.

Pindar introduces us to The Pythia, otherwise known as The Oracle of Delphi, in his poem *Pythian*, from fifth century BCE. *Here, he refers to her* as *Melissa Delphis* – "The Bee of Delphi." Both Euripides and he insist that the priestesses earned their Melissa title because they'd come to be associated with the purity of the bee.[48]

Battus, blessed son of Polymnestus, it was you that, in accord with this word of prophecy, the oracle glorified by the spontaneous cry of the Delphic Bee, who three times loudly bid you hail, and declared that you were the destined king of Cyrene, when you came to ask the oracle what relief the gods would grant you for your stammering voice. And even now, in later days, as in the prime of red-blossoming spring, eighth in the line of Battus' descendants' flourishes Arcesilas.[49]

Revered across the ancient world, The Pythia received questions from visitors and answered in prophetic oracular verse. In a grotto, deep inside the temple, bored out of the mountain's rockface, she sat upon a tripod, above the axis mundi, the omphalos, and dropped her attention down into her womb.

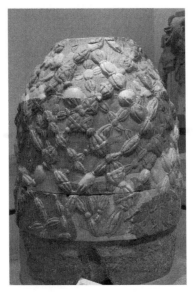

The Omphalos. Photograph by ZDE.

Shaking a laurel branch, she summoned Apollo to speak.

The words of Apollo were drawn up into her grotto from the Earth and pulled up into her vagina as she breathed the pneuma, then circled around the oracular vessel of her womb. In ecstatic trance, she blurted ambiguous sounding verse, always with a 12-beat rhythm to the rhyme.

From 560 BCE to 371 CE, no oracle or diviner was deemed higher. For almost a thousand years, leaders, warriors, and priests came from across the world, to consult the oracle about battle strategies, where to make new settlements and many other questions of state.

Over 500 channelled testimonies of Apollo are recorded, and as Sarah Iles Johnston stated in her essay "Delphia and the Dead", the large percentage of the oracles were from people who wanted to try to contact loved ones who had passed over. Many sources describe the sense of magnetism people experienced as they received their oracles. Others describe some of what happened after they had.

One such tale was of King Croesus who had so much faith in his oracle that he would devote the next decade of his life building the second marvellous incarnation of Artemis' Temple at Ephesus. As stated earlier, Ephesian coins have pictures of bees on them, which is absent in earlier versions, suggesting the symbology may have been a modern introduction perhaps of his invention.[19]

So, how does such deep faith come about? Well, remember that word we shared at the beginning – *epopteia*? To witness. Croesus had witnessed his own inexplicable experience that was to sway him towards his unshakable belief.

We hear how the savvy king established a kind of market research project by despatching emissaries on a 100-day quest to visit the seven most popular oracles. They had a simple objective.

Each must ask the same question of the oracles: "What is Croesus doing today?"

The Oracle of Delphi replied:

I count the grains of sand on the beach and measure the sea; I understand the speech of the dumb and hear the voiceless. The smell has come to my sense of a hard shelled tortoise boiling and bubbling with a lamb's flesh in a bronze pot: the cauldron underneath it is of bronze, and bronze is the lid.

On receiving the oracular replies, Croesus was impressed. Of all of the oracles evaluated, only the Delphic Bee seemed to make any sense. He was shaken by the realisation that he had indeed sat, prepared, and eaten turtle soup, a dish which, he declared, was more suited to peasants than kings. Thus, Croesus sent gold and silver in homage to Delphi, and from that time onwards would consult the oracle many times hence.

The name, Pythia, means "of the python". Mythology tells of how the first oracle was the daughter of Gaia, an enormous pythoness, called Delphyne. Later, another Python, Pytho, was guarding the sanctuary at Delphi, when as we know, he refused to allow Leto to shelter there to deliver her twins. Apollo, in retribution, slayed Pytho and usurped the temple. Traditional bee wisdom says that Pytho, along with Typhon, slithered up and took refuge in the bee skep omphalos. On returning after his exile from Olympia, to atone for this disservice to humanity, he began to breathe wisdom and oracles into the priestesses' vulvae in the form of spirited smoke.

In Homer's *Hymn to Hermes*, we hear Apollo originally learnt the power of divination from the Thriae when they nursed him and taught him their oracular ways.

> *There are certain sacred sisters, three virgins lifted on swift wings; their heads have been dusted with white meal; they live beneath a cliff on Parnassus. They teach their own kind of fortune telling... the sisters fly back and forth from their home, feeding on waxy honeycombs and making things happen. They like to tell the truth when they have eaten honey and the spirit is on them; but if they've been deprived of that divine sweetness, they buzz about, and mumble lies.*
>
> *(Homeric Hymn to Hermes, vv. 552-563)*

These three virginal bee nymphs – also known as Melissae – were Kleodora (meaning "Famed for her Gift"), Daphnis ("Laurel") and Melaina ("The Black").

That they are sisters is engaging, because as we have seen, the priesthoods did seem to draw from certain tribes. Later, we will discover evidence of priestesses with familial links being buried together. Whether the women were *closely* related is uncertain, but there seems to be echoes of the bond found in the sisterhood of the hive.[20]

Bee mistresses, the three Thriae were naiads of the sacred springs at the Corycian Cave of Mount Parnassus.

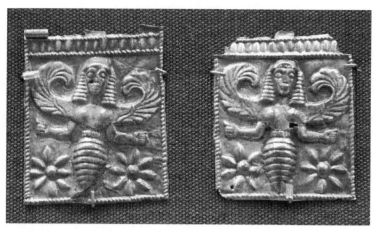

Gold plaques embossed with winged bee goddesses, perhaps the
Thriae, found at Camiros, Rhodes, dated to 7th century BCE,
British Museum.

Daphnis is an interesting name because it links to the laurel in
the Delphic story. There is a myth about how Eros shoots two
arrows in response to Apollo mocking the futility of the way
Eros uses his archer's gift. He shoots a gold arrow at Apollo,
making him fall hopelessly in love with the nymph, Daphne. He
shoots Daphne with a lead one, so she will *hate* Apollo.

Apollo relentlessly pursues Daphne until finally she calls
upon her father to either get rid of the god or change her so that
she can escape him. Oddly, her father decides that it would be
helpful if she were a tree instead, and she becomes a laurel.

I love the idea that maybe the oracle shakes the laurel branch,
and the sacred connection is secretly embodied in the priestess.
It's like this intimate secret hidden from the eyes of men.
Outwardly, they witness the ecstasy, but have no understanding
what mystical union is taking place.

We have two Daphne bushes just down the road from us and
their fragrance, when the sun comes out, is astonishing. The
bush hums with literally hundreds of bees. It happens for just a
few days, somewhere between a week or maybe two. I noticed it

too late to count this year, but next year I shall, and I'm hoping to find that, just like the oracles worked for nine days out of each year, there might be a different nine days where you can predict where all the insect Melissae will be hanging out.

The idea of trees with hundreds of bees in them, and the oracle shaking the laurel, makes me think of how swarms can be shaken from trees. In fact, even the most basic truth that, like the oracles, bees make predictions based on the sun (Apollo)... well, that's *especially* delightful, don't you think? So whimsical, yet such a deeply revered and respectful business.

There's more complex layering to this though, in that an even more ancient spirit guide inhabits the realm, deeper even than the god that the beginnings of patriarchy placed there. For before Apollo drew his sword, mystical serpents ruled this place. The snake might feasibly be the creature who knows most about ambiguity and contradiction, certainly the one who carries most fear with her, and yet such a reputation of power. Consider some of the imagery that accompanies her, and we start to conceive of a far richer understanding of the ecstasy and vision of which the ancient writers reported. With a flicker of her tongue, the serpent can discern whole encyclopaedias of knowledge about what's going on around her. She senses everything through her skin, feeling the very movement of the earth through her belly.

In Hinduism, she represents the power of kundalini, empowered energy rising up the spine with spiritual growth. Poignantly, she shares a certain type of gaze with the oracles, her glassy eyes becoming opaque as if in trance as she sheds her skin. There's a clear correlation between growth and slithering out of her sheath – reminiscent of Inanna shedding her layers of clothing as kundalini grows, shifts, evolves and reveals occult sacred knowledge through many states of consciousness.

The glories of the magnificent Delphi sanctuary have been extolled by many writers over the centuries. It's no wonder the sheer majesty of its location has been such an inspiration. Legends whisper how Zeus, himself, despatched two eagles to show him the most beautiful place on Earth. On setting sight on Parnassus, spellbound, he proclaimed he must make his sanctuary in this place.

Today, conserved as a UNESCO World Heritage Site, the sanctuary at Delphi is one of the most important sites in ancient Greece (second only to the Acropolis). Construction of the sanctuary began in eight century BCE. Temples were dedicated to Apollo and his twin Artemis somewhere around the end of the seventh century BCE, but historically, there are clues that veneration at the site probably stretches back much farther in time. Legends tell how Apollo (or some say Daedalus) fashioned the original temple from beeswax and feathers. Over time, the site grew to include many festivals and games, including the important Pythian Games held every four years to commemorate how Apollo slayed the snake dragon, Delphyne.

You know, if it hadn't been for the wretched virus this year, I think I'd have jumped on a plane to see this place first hand. Reality meant I have had to make do with videos by the British historian, Michael Wood, and a book by an author called William J. Broad. I hesitate to lift text directly from his book, *The Oracle of Delphi*, since it only serves to highlight the inferiority of my own writing skills next to his, but I'll be brave because I'd like you to experience the sanctuary through a first-person account. Broad says:

The most interesting part of my journey began when I finally got to Delphi. It was a revelation. For centuries, writers have struggled to convey its grandeur, describing it as a place where primal forces have thrown open the secrets of the earth to human inquiry. You are enveloped by mountains and canyons and cliffs and slopes that stretch out in a staggering array of hues and removes, some lush and intimate, some cool and faraway, so that every time you walk around a little bit or turn your head, you glimpse a hidden world or, across a wider expanse, a striking new view. It's like having your favorite sights from a lifetime of hiking all gathered into one spot. Sound reinforces the splendor. Close your eyes intermittently and you can better appreciate the song of the wind, of crickets, of water on rock, of sheep in pasture, of bees in almond blossoms. One day while climbing the surrounding hills I came upon a herd of migrating goats. Their bells captivated me with the syncopated clang of metal on metal and the thump of wood on wood.

(See my hesitation? Man, that man can write! I think I'll just give up and go home!)

As you reached Delphi on the approach to Parnassus, the temple was hidden, but as you rounded the ravine you would have been met by the most opulent displays of wealth. Statues and offerings from state leaders who had wanted to express their thanks surrounded the temple on every side. Smaller temples and annexes made of gold and precious stones reflected the light conveying opulence, and a tremendously lengthy wait between you and your question. Hundreds of querents queued to ask for help with decisions every scheduled prophecy day.

I love to imagine the soundscape not just of Broad's goats and crickets, but of bags being dumped on the floor, the wonder of arriving, fading to exasperation of the wait. The jibber jabber of Babel as hundreds of tongues uttered their news, their questions, and details of the journey they had undertaken.

I wonder, how much did they reveal about the question that had demanded this slog?

As they marvelled at each new piece of art, prime examples of their time, how much did that contribute to their assurance that their quest was sane.

Outside on the walls, graffiti extolled thousands of words of gratitude for favour bestowed by Melissa.

When finally, they reached the front of the queue, a lintel graced the door above their heads. *"Know thyself,"* it said. Another, originating from a separate doorway, reminded the visitor, *"Everything in moderation."*

Originally, Melissa Delphis had only channelled Apollo once a year, but at the height of her fame, there were three Melissae working a shift system. The oracle would be available for consultation nine months a year, giving prophesies on the seventh day following the new moon. Unlike other priesthoods, the role was not inherited. Rather, the priestess was chosen by election from the community.

Greek mythology describes how the position of the oracle had initially been held by maidens, but after a horrific incident when Echekrates had raped one of the young women, rules had had to be adapted. From that time on, the Pythia would only ever be chosen from women over 50. To commemorate those early younger priestesses, the older women continued to wear the maiden's garb.

To cleanse herself for communion with the god, Melissa Delphis bathed in the Kastalian Spring. Then, according to tradition, the words of Apollo were visited upon her through hallucinogenic volcanic fumes seeping up through a floor of the spring.

After sacrificing a goat, she descended into the *adyton*, her sacred inner sanctum located beneath the temple. Plutarch tells how she made offerings of barley meal and laurel onto the altar, before climbing upon the great bronze tripod that had been made for her. There, over the omphalos, the navel of the Earth and focal point of the temple, she rhythmically shook her laurel and waited for the god to speak.

Orgasmic in trance, Melissa Delphis pronounced judgement and prophecy for her querents who, in readiness, had paid their fee to the priestess and sacrificed their own laurel and black rams, in the hope that Apollo might see fit to offer counsel.

If you want to learn more about the Oracle at Delphi, I can heartily recommend the book the Parnassus description comes from. Broad is a Pulitzer Prize-winning journalist. His prose reads like lustrous velvet; his research is unrelenting. I salivated at every word.

His book tells the true story of a geologist and fanatical classicist, who observes something about the site that no-one ever has before – or actually, they had, but had ignored it not understanding its relevance – an enormous crack that betrayed the site sitting right over a geological fault.

Not long after discovering it, he meets an archaeologist who scoffs at his thoughts knowing of lengthy excavations done by the French where nothing of the priestess' chamber, the *adyton*, had been found.

What the geologist de Boer hadn't known was that, for many years, by then, the Pythia had been dismissed and accepted as probably nothing more than the stuff of legend. Eyewitness accounts had been discounted since French archaeologist, Théophile Homolle, had led a large team in long and rigorous excavations in 1892, but failed to find the chasm.

The book tells of de Boer and Hale's wonderful joint intelligence of understanding different things, then when they added more scholars with equally disparate knowledge, it brought a new picture into being. I have to say, as an aromatherapist trying to find things Greek scholars had never been able to, I found it most heartening.

Spoiler alert... Eventually their findings lead them to the discovery that ethylene would have seeped into the grotto, a gas widely recognised as hallucinogenic.

Now, to be clear, I loved every space, comma, and carefully placed word in this book. I adored the vivid pictures he painted of the surrounding landscape and the way I felt empowered by understanding each newly-discovered piece of science. I held my breath at each hypothesis and actually made the family jump out of their TV reverie, whooping, when one of their test results finally came back confirmed.

I cannot recommend the book highly enough to you.

But at the end, I was left cold and more than a little irritated.

I found it fascinating then, that the author concluded the book by admitting that both he and de Boer had felt the same emptiness I had, when the world was satisfied that the hallucinogen was the whole tale.

Because to put a millennium's worth of celebrity down to nothing more than being high, takes away the women's power. It implies they spoke nothing more than gibberish, but if that were true, what does that say about all the graffiti, all that gratitude from people who felt the oracles had helped them? Those words would make no sense unless their writers felt the transaction that took place had been anything but real.

To suggest these oracles were "just women, uttering unintelligible symbols to be then transcribed and translated by men" most *definitely* takes away their power. What was it about being priestly that provided insights? How utterly patronising to suggest they could construe what the priestess could not.

To insinuate that there were spies amongst the throngs, inhabiting inns and restaurants gathering gossip and clues to inform details of the oracular utterances... takes away their power.

Because it *has* been assumed that the agency of the prophetess herself has been exaggerated or invented. How could a local woman, elected by the people, have dispensed advice on such complex political issues as colonisation and tyranny, they say.

Associate Professor of Classical and Medieval Studies at Bates College in Maine, Lisa Maurizio, echoes my fury arguing "to deny the Pythia her agency in this religious rite is to render the spectacle of consulting Apollo incomprehensible."

It's true, isn't it?

Why would anyone ask for Apollo's advice if the women were frauds? How could something endure for centuries if people gained no merit from it? Most of all, how could it have become such a phenomenon in a civilization that is recognised as one of the most respected of all time? It makes no sense.

Maurizio's argument strengthens, as she examines terminology and language used. An overlap appearing around the Melissae Delphis and the priests supporting them fascinates her.

Mantis – the word for seer – derives from the root word meaning *men*, but just as often it alludes to altered mental states we might call inspiration.

Phophetes – originates from the word "to say" or "to speak". It means someone who proclaims publicly.

For a long time, traditional thinking described Melissa offering inspiration, in utterances, as *mantis*. The *prophetai* were then seen as stepping in to make sense of the babble and writing it down to submit it to record.

But on close examination of contemporary texts surrounding them, the oracle might be referred to as *mantis*, but just as regularly, as *phophetis* and even *pro-mantis* which would dub her "fore-seer".

(Likewise, I wonder, if their functions were priestly, whether we should also interpret them as being, in some way, Praying Mantis?)

A cauldron of so many roles and meanings all rolled into one.

Breton Connelly, in *Portrait of a Priestess*, powerfully illustrates the agency of the Pythia, as a forceful and authoritative presence. These examples feel at odds with the idea of a subordinate sanctuary servant.

She relates how, on one occasion, despite it being considered inauspicious for prophecies to take place on any other day but the seventh after certain new moons, one Phoenician leader, Philomelos, didn't have the patience to wait for his.

He seized control of Delphi, in 356 BCE, and ordered the Pythia to climb on her tripod according to the custom. When she bit back, correcting that, actually, it *wasn't* the custom, he resorted to threats. Unperturbed the Melissa replied coolly: "It is in your power to do as you please." On imagining he had finally forced her into giving him his oracle, he was placated. He took the words as confirmation that he should continue to conduct his military plans. Two years later at the Battle of Neon, his prophecy was to take a darker turn. The Boeotians, furious for his overthrow of Delphi, slaughtered him in vengeance for his acts.

The famous general and historian, Xenophon, described that on one occasion, one pious pilgrim asked for advice about how best to please the gods. I have to say I was impressed by such an interesting question, but apparently, it wasn't an unusual one, and that the oracle's answer would always be the same. The most righteous approach was to revere the local customs of one's own state and nation, and to honour their indigenous deities and spirits. At the beginning of this research, I found that an extremely disconcerting statement; a woman who lives on the border of the Land of the Druids, seeking to know Grecian gods. By the end though, it simply makes me smile and I now find I completely concur.

Aristexonos reported that one Delphic Priestess, Themistokleia, schooled an incredibly famous student, none other than Pythagoras. Indeed, we learn from Pythagoras' biography, written by Iamblichus in the second century CE, that his very birth had been predicted when his own father had consulted the Pythia and she, in turn, had told him he was to have an extraordinary son. Iamblicus points out that his very name Pythagoras originates from Pythia.

I will stress that my son, who is a maths scholar, argues that almost everything we know about Pythagoras is myth, but I can't help but ponder on this reputed training, and the detail that he and his disciples were believed to have venerated the honeycomb shape of the hexagon as divine.

One of my personal favourite stories of the oracle is that someone is reputed to have asked her who was the wisest person in the world. The Pythia gave Socrates' name. When quizzed about it later, he replied: "One thing I know, is that I know nothing."

Indeed, Socrates was fascinated by this very truth. It was to become a deep sense of purpose in his years to come. He took to asking questions in a particular way, to try to identify and pinpoint truth.

The technique involves rigorous questioning, over and over, to assess a person's hypothesis, until it inevitably ends up revealing a contradiction. The Socratic Method of Learning remains one of philosophy's most important tools. Viewed as an invaluable method to ensure critical thinking, it is still used to train lawyers *par excellence* today.

Socrates was fascinated with paradoxes and contradictions, eh? And the Pythia thought that was wise. Yes, I am fairly certain a Melissa probably would.

Three thousand years from her first utterance, her final words are preserved.

Tell the emperor that my hall has fallen to the ground. Phoibos no longer has his house, nor his mantic bay, nor his prophetic spring; the water has dried up.

Although, in *Delphic Oracle: Its Responses and Operations*, Joseph Fontenrose is not convinced. He feels the quotation reeks of Christian bias, carefully constructed to suggest that the Messiah's coming now made the oracles redundant, and that it *must* have been right and true, because the oracles themselves had foretold it.

Over, their days may be, but gone, they are not.

Preserved in our collective memory and kept safe in no lesser place than Vatican City. They have pride of place, in the glorious majesty of the Sistine Chapel. They occupy all four corners of Michelangelo's frieze, overseeing the miraculous transaction of God, bearing witness to the conception of the Christ-child.

Chapter 12

Aphrodite

Perhaps the image that best serves the bee priestesses is as servants of Aphrodite; bees blissfully producing golden nectar of the gods. The Greeks called bees the birds of the muses, as such they inspired music, and the very expression of beauty through art and poetry. The Greek concept of beauty, "kallos" possessed a far more sophisticated meaning than it does today. Rather than just the notion of an attractive physical body, beauty combined with virtues of the soul. Honey and the hive were metaphors for sweetness and service to something bigger, the service of love. All of these were considered to be beauteous aspects of sacred femininity and the priestesshood.

Scholars believe the foundation site of the cult of Aphrodite was probably the Minoan colony at Cythera. However, legend tells that she was born on Aphrodite's Rock, just offshore of the road between Paphos and Limassol in Cyprus. Here, sapphire blue skies kissed grain-coloured rocks and it really wouldn't be hard to imagine her emerging from the sparkling waters of this place. Indeed, Homer calls her The Cyprian and her most important sanctuaries were found at Paphos and Amathus there.

On the Greek mainland, she was worshipped in Athens and at the east end of the Gulf of Corinth, about 50 miles west of Athens.

Her symbols are the swallow, sparrow, dolphin, swan, pearl, mirror, scallop shell, the apple, and the dove. The dove, the sparrow and the swan are said to be her sacred animals.

Her origin myth is perhaps most famously depicted in Botticelli's painting of the *Birth of Venus* but the story of what came before the beautiful Goddess in her shell is, really, quite something.

Gaia, sick to the back teeth of being persistently pregnant by her husband-son Ouranos, decided to take matters into her own hands. Taking another of her sons, Cronus, aside, she tried to persuade him to do something about his dad. Cronus fashioned himself a sickle from a jagged flint and hacked his father's solid rutting phallus off, slinging the penis and testicles into the briny sea.

The waves collided. Blood and semen mixed, and from the gory froth, rose an "awful and lovely maiden". The name Aphrodite literally means: "She who rose from the foam."

The seismic wave swells into magnificent goriness. It edges its way onto the shore and then the land. As she reaches the sand, she moves across the dusty plains shooting greenery and flowers from beneath her feet as her moistness plunges into the soil. I love to think of the bees following close behind, buzzing around her sweetness, and dancing on these newly sprung blooms. Birds sing in the trees and the air becomes noisy with the sound of frogs and toads. Born from violence and rage, the goddess is the fecund incarnation of life cycles, and the manifestation of life itself.

Aphrodite has close associations with several other mythological entities. Notably, with Eros, the god of desire, with the Charites (known by the Romans as The Graces), and the Horae who were personifications of the seasons. Through these, she is emphasised as a promoter of fertility but also, like Persephone, she is seen as The Goddess Of Spring. (Her sacred month is April.)

The poet Lucretius perhaps most gloriously captured the magnificence of Aphrodite when he called her "Genetrix" – the *Creative Element of the World*. Here, we might think of butterflies on flowers, but also inspiration, glorious artworks, melodious tunes, sumptuous fabrics... the list goes on.

Genetrix – she who generates...

Yet, The Goddess Of Love being in some way connected to the way bees pollinate is rather curious, since history gives no indication that the Greeks had any understanding of how *human* fertilisation took place. Indeed, the nuts and bolts of how eggs and sperm combine to make babies wasn't discovered until the 17th century CE, and even then, knowledge was cursory. Nevertheless, the whispered oral tradition is clear. A Melissa priestess could control if a sperm met her egg.

The Goddess has many names, but two main epithets: *Ourania* and *Pandemos*. *Aphrodite Ourania*, meaning *"Heavenly Dweller"* may relate to her astrological association with Venus and is thought to be her older manifestation. Here she was imagined as the child of Zeus and Dione, the presiding Goddess of the oracular site, Dodona.

Most often, The Goddess is referred to as *Aphrodite Pandemos* meaning *"Common to All People"*. The most technical translation of her name means "within the city state" which Plato, in *Symposium*, revealed was a reference to **intellectual and common love**.

Other names offer more clues of how she was conceived in people's minds:

In his First Hymn to Aphrodite, Homer calls her *Philommeidés* (φιλομμειδής) – "smile-loving".[50] This is generally accepted as meaning "laughter-loving".[52] Although, Monica Cyrino, Professor of Classics at the University of New Mexico says that when Hesiod calls her *Philommeidés* in Theogony the interpretation seems closer to "genital-loving", than smile loving.

Strangely, for a goddess known for being so lovely, for a long time, she wasn't really depicted as anything special. Legend says that around the fourth century BCE, the island of Kos commissioned the sculptor, Praxiteles, to make them an image of Aphrodite. He did. In fact, he sculpted two. One where she was fully clothed and another magnificent image of the goddess of beauty entirely naked.

The statue shocked the inhabitants of Kos. They were outraged that he could have done such a disrespectful thing. It was unheard of for a woman to be sculpted nude, let alone someone as venerated as a goddess, and they railed against the carving. The nearby islanders of Knidos got wind of the beautiful artistry going cheap, so they snatched up the bargain and placed it in the sanctuary of Aphrodite at Knidos.

The Aphrodite of Knidos was quite the tourist attraction and sailors, in particular, were drawn to the temple. Each stood before her mesmerised by her winsome grace. One tale tells of how a sailor could not get her image out of his mind and he snuck into the temple in the dead of night, just to gaze a little longer upon her. But it was too much. He was unable to contain himself and left a most inappropriate stain on her thigh.

Artists tell of what a beguiling tease the statue was. One hand resting on her bathrobe and the other coyly protecting her genitalia, her modesty paradoxically drawing the eye. Over the centuries, this would come to be a common theme of Aphrodite's: clothed, but not clothed; coy and yet utterly seductive. It was this statue that functioned as muse for the *Venus de Milo* now on permanent display in the Louvre. Sadly, the original Aphrodite of Knidos was lost, perhaps in a fire in 476 CE.

One might say that Aphrodite Pandemos enjoys two births, the mythical one by Ouranus and another more historical one, where she developed from the Mother Goddess of Anatolia, Mesopotamia, and the Levant.

Earlier we spoke of Venus statuettes. Cyprus had their own strange version of these. Dating from around 3000 BCE and usually made from the beautiful soft, bluey green stone, pectolite, these strange figures have been found right across Cyprus, but mainly down its south-western side. Again, the Goddess has lusciously fleshy thighs and oversized breasts and sex – but this time their arms are stretched out to the sides and their heads are moulded into a graphic depiction of a phallus.

The effect is cruciform, and probably shows the still-used birthing position of a woman being supported in her squatting labour from behind.[51]

Two larger versions of these have been found, which measure about 30cm tall, but most are very tiny, with holes punched into their tops as if they have been worn as amulets. It's thought the larger ones might be cultic figures, and the smaller ones, more personal, portable depictions of those. The majority of the amulet figures have been unearthed from children's graves. When found in adults' tombs, they mostly seem to have belonged to women. Scholars suggest the amulets may have been worn to bless their pregnancies or perhaps even worn in the hope of conceiving, promoting its likelihood using some kind of sympathetic magic.[51]

This sympathy is an interesting notion that tells us much about the figurines found in temples too. Rather like we view icons today, as somewhat different from your everyday picture – that somehow they *embody* the Virgin and Christ – so, we should consider these statuettes as embodiments of divinity too. The Venus amulet was fertility hanging around the supplicant's neck.

Interestingly, some of these figurines have been found with their own amulets hanging around *their* necks too, perhaps a depiction of how life perpetuates on and on. These figurines might have protected homes or spoken of the love a woman has for her child, or even the regenerative nature of sex, but not yet really any sense of romantic love.

The name Aphrodite doesn't appear in Cyprus until the fifth century BCE when Greek influence begins to take hold. Inscriptions in the sixth century BCE are dedicated to "the Wanassa".

Wanassa is the feminine form of the Greek word **Anax** (Greek: Ἄναξ; from earlier Ϝάναξ, wánax) that means "tribal chief, lord, (military) leader".[52]

The Wanassa was a female tribal leader – the sovereign. She was a war queen and a fertility Goddess whose fetish was fragranced oils. As the Eastern war Goddess merged with the local goddess of fertility, we see the face of Aphrodite starting to appear.[53]

This goddess of murderous warmongering and lascivious urges is the beginnings of the ancestors of Aphrodite. The goddesses of love and war, Inanna, Ishtar and Astarte were all said to draw their powers from the planet Venus, a star of most unpredictable habits.[27] Understood, long ago, to be two planets – the morning and evening stars – Venus meandered across the skies in a fickle manner, bewildering all who watched. Is it any wonder she struck terror into the hearts of men?

In her book, *Venus and Aphrodite*, Bettany Hughes tells us that the Neo-Assyrian King of Nineveh, in 680 BCE, cursed a group of traitors of his court, declaring:

May Venus, the brightest of the stars, before your eyes make your wives lie in the laps of your enemy.[27]

Terrifying she may have been, but the Eastern Goddess was worshipped devoutly. It is believed that in Babylon alone, Inanna had more than 180 sanctuaries dedicated to her. Located in Mesopotamia, about 60 miles south of Baghdad, in modern-day Iraq, Babylon marked the beginning of the Silk Routes. The stronghold possessed the perfect qualities to spread the seed of the fertility Goddess far and wide. Indeed, we know from the *Epic of Gilgamesh* that the Temple of Ishtar was a bustling worship centre where hundreds of merchants also networked daily, exchanging news and contemporary ideas alongside the goods they traded. Spice laden ships brought incense and perfumes to Cyprus' shore and took away fruits, ivory, amber and metals. Many ships would arrive simply to buy Cyprus' copper, a vital component of bronze weaponry manufacture.

That copper, then, fell under the arbitration of the priestess of Aphrodite gives galvanising insights into her power.

Just as the fetish of Wanassa was scented oils, so Aphrodite was always described as sweetly and being bathed by The Graces in perfume.

The smoking altar. That blissful fragrance, so irresistible to the bee Goddess, swirling around her as oils are rubbed all over her by her attendants. (Don't forget how the queen bee is fed and cared for by the youngest nurse bees, and we see the smoke going in to calm and please her...)

I have this prevailing image of the woman, stood before the altar. Potentially, like Gaia, so completely over being pregnant all the time, charged with the responsibility of populating the polis, and sensing this deep erotic love. And in that moment, rather than reaching for a kiss from her lover, she reaches for something charged with beauty. Whether she channels that ardour into arranging flowers, embroidering, dancing, writing, singing, or simply entering her own reverie... the communion with Aphrodite opens. Allowing spirit to move through her, to move and inform the reawakening of her soul and her rawness. In Melissa terms, this is known as impersonal sex. Every action done from the heart, brings her closer to the realm of nature and her spirits. Explored from that angle, the depictions on the Minoan seals positively drip honey from how dazzling the priestesses felt, transformed, ethereal and ecstatic.

And I can't help but connect that with the statuettes of Venus, and how they seemed to have controlled their births somehow. Pregnancy on her terms, if and when she wanted it.[54]

So, I'm really feeling this vibration, you know. The buzz feels right. I can sense the resonance of the lesson, but something feels very, very *wrong*, and that is that followers of Aphrodite are not usually referred to as bees... they are doves. Nevertheless, there are so many Internet pages, particularly on Pinterest (but not many places of scholastic note, I will admit), that say the priestesses of Aphrodite at Eryx were Melissae.

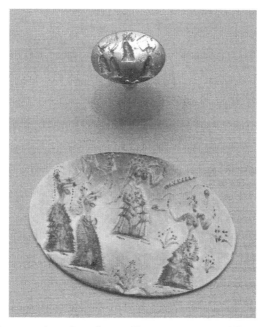

Minoan Isopata ring, found near Knossos. Late middle II Kingdom,
c. 1500 BCE. Photograph by Olaf Tausch.

Specifically, Eryx.

That's interesting, or it would be if I could find it in the primary sources, but I can't. I can't even find it written in any academic papers.

The same few facts keep coming up thus:

Melissae would lay honeycombs onto the altar of Aphrodite at Mt. Eryx where The Goddess' fetish was a honeycomb, and that there was a honeycomb that had been fashioned out of gold by Daedalus.

My lovely friend Lori Glenn, Managing Director of HerbalGram, who has made a lifelong study of the Sicilian stories of Aphrodite, told me that Sicily has black bees. Close cousins of African bees, they are known for their gentleness and calm. It's probable that women working with them wouldn't have needed a veil, conjuring pictures of those bare-breasted priestesses, hearts open, vulnerable, and exposed, wearing nothing else but those spectacular skirts.[55]

Aphrodite's temple at Eryx sat high on the mountainside of the Sicilian coast and was the first thing sailors saw as they approached from Africa. Ancient sources tell us that after climbing the steep cliff face, sailors would enter the temple and participate in sacred sexual fertility rites with the priestess standing in proxy of The Goddess. The same was said of the goddess' sanctuary at Corinth.

But, whilst priestesses at Eryx seemed to be famous in their own right, I found no ancient sources describing them as Melissae, or bees. Most referred to them as "Jerodulai".

When I put that into Google Translate, Italian to English, it churned out "Hiero doula". Not a word, but certainly, a notion of something. That thing being sacred servant. That would certainly be coherent as Melissa. But the ancient Greek noun doulē actually means female *slave*, and this seems to possess a darker connotation. Not because of the sex *per se*, because while a woman can have relations with whomever she chooses to my mind, the *agency* of the priestess seems to be in question here. In fact, it's the choosing that's the issue. There seems to be a suggestion of force, and that stopped me in my tracks.

It doesn't feel right at all.

We think of The Delphic oracles, how strong they had to be against political leaders. Likewise, other priestesses were powerful decision makers in charge of huge amounts of wealth. A Melissa is not a wallflower. She is a bee and bees have stings.

Nope. I'm sorry. It just doesn't feel right.

Not least because there seems to be so little parity between the duties of the priestesses at different cult centres. When a young woman was about to wed, for example, and wanted to ask for help being a successful wife, replete with fertility, she first visited the Temple of Artemis to bid farewell to the goddess who had supported her in her formative years and then went to

Aphrodite's temple in Athens to ask her to now take over the favour.

In comparison to the sacred sex with sailors at Eryx then, Athens must have felt very tame. The chasms between the expectations seem too large.

Except, then I found out the Athenian temple was paid for by a magistrate who funded it with his takings from his club that ran male sex workers. It's not feeling very romantic at all. Perhaps we have not got Aphrodite quite right.

Maybe if we go further back in time?

Aphrodite and Adonis

Her most famous myth, after her origins story, is arguably the tale of her love of Adonis and the dreadful pact she had to make with Persephone. It's a complex myth, of taboo desires, sophisticated attractions and difficult relationships that can never end well. At a deeper level, though, you can see themes of seasonal changes and the moral that no matter how dark the days are, spring will eventually come, but Aphrodite's neglect of her duties as Theia, in her lovesick following of Adonis in the forest, is a perfect metaphor for the way we experience life on Earth changing when Venus starts to retrograde.

Of course, then he gets gored by the boar, so it's bye-bye Adonis.

Sobbing on the floor, cradling his corpse, Aphrodite's tears fell and mingled with his blood and an anemone sprang from the union. (Or some say it was a white rose and her blood turned it red.)

In her grief, Aphrodite carried a cypress branch with her, as a constant reminder of her mourning, and decreed that all women, every summer, should celebrate a memorial of Adonis' life, the Adonia. Until recently it was thought that Adonia took place at the summer solstice, but in 2003, Dillon suggested a likelier scenario may have been that the women grieved him in spring. They planted lettuce and fennel in shallow terracotta pots and placed them onto their roofs to grow in the midday heat.

The fast-growing salad leaves would shoot but then, frazzled by the sun and unable to root, they quickly withered and died. At that, the women would publicly tear their clothes and beat their breasts in mourning for the goddess' beloved, Adonis. Interestingly, this was a public ceremony, orchestrated by the women themselves, rather than a state officiated ritual.

As is often the case with religious myths, the story of Aphrodite and Adonis is not new.

It is thought that whilst Aphrodite is believed to have originated in Cyprus, Adonis came later, from the Near East. His name derives from a Canaanite word meaning Lord. The myth reflects an earlier Babylonian story of Inanna and Dumuzid or their Semitic counterparts, Ishtar and Tammuz, which is recounted in the Old Testament book of Ezekiel 8:14 where the women mourn the passing of Tammuz at the North Gate of the Temple of Jerusalem. The cult of Adonis seems to have been associated with the Phoenician cult of Ba'al.

In *Greek Religion*, Walter Burkert relates:

Women sit by the gate weeping for Tammuz, or they offer incense on roof-tops and plant pleasant plants. These are the very features of the Adonis legend: which is celebrated on flat roof-tops on which sherds sown with quickly germinating green salading are placed, Adonis gardens... the climax is loud lamentation for the dead god.[22]

Interpretatio graeco is work done by the ancient Greeks themselves to try to bring some cohesion and to understand relationships between beliefs of different cultures. This chart pulls some of the archetypes together for us.

Greek (Romanised)	Adonis
Etruscan	Atunis
Egyptian	Osiris
Sumerian	Dumuzid
Phoenician	Adōn/Tammuz

As already stated, the traditional symbol of Aphrodite isn't a bee. It's a dove.

This originated from a syncretism from another Goddess by the name of Semiramis, whose myths are likely based on the true life story of an Assyrian warrior queen from the first millennium BCE.

The most famous myth about Semiramis is told by Diodorus Siculo, but other tales about her arise in works by Plutarch, Justinius, Eusebius and Polybius. She is a well-documented goddess, but it's likely her tales were inspired by the life of the real queen Shammu-ramat, a queen regent of the Assyrian Empire.

When her husband died, she continued to reign in place of her son until he came of age. She is recorded as having reigned between 811-806 BCE.

In the origin myth of Semiramis, according to Diodorus, she was the daughter born of a mortal man and the fish goddess of wisdom, Derketo. The pregnancy was the result of some tragic union. (I can't remember what... it's probably relevant but there's no need to complicate the tale...)

After the birth, Derketo drowned herself, abandoning the child to raise herself alone. Doves found her and began to feed her, continuing to do so until she was found by a royal shepherd, entirely covered by beautiful white birds, and was taken back to court. There she grew, was wooed, married a general, came into her mother's powers of wisdom and offered useful advice and strategies of how to wage war. Eventually, so respected was she, that she was even able to lead her own soldiers into battle.

The inevitable happened, of course. Beautiful, powerful woman. Can't be left alone. The king decided that, even though she and the general seemed to be extremely happy, he had to have her. He offered the general money, who politely declined. The jealous king then pulled his ace card, threatening to gouge out the general's eyes. That seems to have done the trick. Semiramis was taken to the palace.

So, the king married Semiramis. They had a fruitful marriage and she bore a son. Years later though, the king was killed by an arrow in battle, so sensing the danger of a power vacuum, Semiramis disguised herself as the new heir, her now fully-grown son. The soldiers, wishing to obey their new king, unwittingly heeded her commands and Semiramis led the nation to a powerful victory.

What's perhaps interesting here is how she was able to disguise herself so convincingly as her son, because as I said at the beginning, Melissa teachings say that most powerful of the priestesses, the ones who have gained control of their necktary, are said to be able to shapeshift. Eventually, their glands were said to have begun to secrete ichor, the blood of the gods.

The real queen Shammu-ramat must have been quite something to have been the inspiration for the myths of a goddess like this. I can't imagine the Assyrians were an easy nation to rule, for anyone, but especially when rulership by a woman was so unusual. The story says that after King Ninus' death, she reigned for 42 years, conquered great swathes of Asia, rebuilt the great Babylon, and built an enormous wall around the city.

This story by Diodorus is quite a late one but Semiramis had been aligned with The Goddesses Ishtar and Astarte long before he wrote it. Inanna, Astarte, and Ishtar, whilst being goddesses of love, fertility, and procreation, were also goddesses of war, just as Cybele had been, and like her, each carried the epithet, Queen of Heaven.

Now, we have two solid authorities that inform us that Semiramis can, at least in one aspect, be identified with the Assyrian Goddess, or Astarte. These are Athenagoras, an Athenian Christian philosopher from the second century CE,[56] and Lucian, in his famous work, *De Dea Syria*,[10] which translates to "On the Assyrian Goddess" and was also written in the second century CE.

The name "Astarte" also dubs her Cybele or Rhea. In Ovid's work *Opera* he calls Her: "the tower-bearing Goddess" that "made (towers) in cities."[57]

In *Nineveh and Its Remains*, Austen Henry Layard also mentions that in the Syrian Temple of Hierapolis, "She [the Syrian Goddess] was represented as standing on a lion crowned with towers." Again, also symbols of Cybele.

The name, "Asht-tart", actually means "The woman that made towers". There is lots of etymological evidence that "Tart" comes from the verb Tr meaning "to surround" or "encompass", which the word "Tor" also comes from.[58]

In that guise, we might also see another name of the Queen of Heaven – Ashtoreth – who was the goddess said to have built a great wall. In the future, the Magdalene would also come to be known as The Tower.

Let's revisit the idea of Semiramis being Astarte, but also being a dove. Now, the symbol of the dove becomes Astarte, the mother of the world, and the manifestation of the divine feminine. She is the spirit of The Goddess.

As contemporary readers, you and I might consider the way the dove appears as the living embodiment of the Holy Spirit, descending into Jesus at his baptism, in the New Testament, but how it also appears in the story of Noah and the Flood.

The Genesis flood story is thought to derive from the *Epic of Gilgamesh*, far older, dating to the second millennium BCE. In that context, we see the Babylonian divine feminine – Astarte – landing as a dove, redressing the balance of the wrath of the masculine force of the deity, Ea and mediating humankind's healing through the protagonist of the story, Utnapishtim. The same happens with Noah, of course.

The dove and water are connected.

Semiramis then, worshiped as a dove, is regarded as the incarnation of the Holy Spirit. The dove is the bee that the Egyptians worshipped as Ka.

The next part is lifted, almost word for word, from an 1862 book called *The Two Babylons, Or The Papal Worship Proved to Be The Worship of Nimrod and His Wife*.[58] It's written by a Scottish church minister from Arbroath. Those of you familiar with Arbroath, will likely conjure the notion of clever hours in front of the fire, because it's too ruddy cold to do anything else! There must be years of thoughts and research in this section, and I can't help but wonder if its writer the Rev. Alexander Hislop might perhaps also have had bees. Some of the places he looked for backup in his research are incredibly arcane. I wonder how else he might have thought of to check them!

His book, *The Two Babylons*, posits that the Roman Catholic religion, in its entirety, can be traced back directly to worship of the Mesopotamian god, Nimrod, at the city of Nineveh, an important trading point on the Tigris, now found in modern-day Iraq.

He relates that according to the Latin writer Lucius Ampelius,[59] Semiramis, deified as Dove, signifies to us the more gracious and benign aspects of Astarte.

He calls her, *"Deam benignam et misericordem hominibus ad vitam bonam,"* that is "The Goddess benignant and merciful to men" (bringing them) "to a good and happy life."

This benign aspect of her character has two different names attached to it. These are Aphrodite and Mylitta.

Aphrodite, he explains, holds the epithet of mediatrix.

In this guise of mediatrix, Aphrodite is considered "The wrath-sub-duer".[58]

The second term, Mylitta, is a Greek word that means the same.

Mylitta means "Mediatrix".

Are you keeping up? Because now it's going to get clever...

Actually, just do me a favour, would you?

Say them aloud for a minute, as we go...

Aphrodite...

Mylitta

The Hebrew word **Melitz** appears in Job 33. Our English translation is:

> *If there be a messenger with him, an interpreter, one among a thousand, to shew unto man his uprightness.*

Melitz = Messenger or interpreter.

Now translate that into the ancient Turkish dialect of Chaldee...

C'mon, hurry up...

What? You didn't study Chaldee at school? Blimey, kids of today. What do they teach them?

Please. Allow me...

Melitz translated into Chaldee becomes **Melitt**.

Are you still saying it aloud... have you got it yet? Are you feeling the knowing?

Melitz "the messenger, the interpreter", who is a mediator; and "gracious" to men.

The Hebrew and English Lexicon by John Pankhurst, derives this word **"Melitz"** from **"Mltz"**, the masculine declination of the verb "to be sweet", its feminine counterpart being **Melitza**, from which comes **Melissa**, a "bee".

In his words:

Melissa, a common name of the priestesses of Cybele, and as we may infer of Cybele, as Astarte, or Queen of Heaven, herself; for, after Porphyry, has stated that "the ancients called the priestesses of Demeter, Melissae," he adds, that they also "called the Moon Melissa" (Deantro Nympharum, p. 18).

We have evidence, further, that goes to identify this title as a title of Semiramis. Melissa or Melitta (*Apollodorus*, **vol. i. lib. ii., p. 110**) – for the name is given in both ways – is said to have been the mother of Phoroneus, the first that reigned, in whose days the dispersion of mankind occurred, divisions having come in among them, whereas before, all had been in harmony and spoke one language (*Hyginus*, **fab. 143, p. 114**).

Clearly, the tower of Babel, and he concludes the section by summing up the symbol of the Dove for us, and by extension, the name and symbol of Melissa.

in other words, as the woman in whom the "Spirit of God" was incarnate; and thus, appeared as the "Dea Benigna," "The Mediatrix" for sinful mortals. The first form of Astarte, as Eve, brought sin into the world; the second form before the Flood, was avenging as The Goddess Of Justice. This form was "Benignant and Merciful." Thus, also Semiramis, or Astarte, as Venus The Goddess Of Love And Beauty, became "The hope of the whole world," and men gladly had recourse to the "mediation" of one so tolerant of son.

God bless the Reverend and all who sail in him... what a tremendous piece of work. A very clever man.

In a fragment of Orphic poetry, quoted by Natalie Comes, *Melitta* is spoken of as a hive, and given the name called Seira, or the hive of Venus:

Let us celebrate the hive of Venus, who rose from the sea: that hive of many names: the mighty fountain, from whence all kings are descended; from whence all the winged and immortal Loves were again produced.

Hesychius is adamant that the word Seira had several interpretations, amongst which were *Melitta*, which could mean bee, hive, or house of *Melitta*.

Historian Jacob Bryant wrote in *A New System, or, an Analysis of Ancient Mythology*:

[she] was thus represented in ancient mythology, as being the receptacle, from whence issued that swarm, by which the world was peopled.

Reverend Hislop says that Seira was none other than Demeter, the supposed mother of mankind, who was *also* styled as Melitta and Melissa, and was viewed as the Venus of the East. This Deity, *Melitta*, was the same as *Mylitta*, the well-known Venus of the Babylonians and Arabians.

Melitta is also said to be the mother-wife of Phoroneus, son of the river god Inachus. Mythologically, Inachus was known as "the first that reigned"; it was said that in his days the dispersion of mankind occurred. Prior to that, all had harmoniously spoken one language. This too concurs with Reverend Hislop's argument. Melitta, it was said, was a Melia.

So, we have come full circle, back to those original Meliades again. Those spirits that inhabit ash trees and the *M. officinalis* plant. But to evaluate to see how much you have been listening at the back...

Can you remember how these Meliades were supposed to have originated?

I wrote: *According to the poet, Hesiod, Meliades were the very first Melissae, born from droplets of blood that fell onto Gaia, when Ouranus was castrated by his son, Cronus.*

Context is a wonderful thing, isn't it? It's the same origin story as Aphrodite's. The goddess of love and beauty was born from the drops of her father's blood in the water, and the Meliades, when they fell upon the Earth. There is the split again. This time, not love and war, or East and West, but divinity ruling Earth, water and, of course, because The Goddess is a bee, the air. In the middle, stands the Mediatrix – Melissa, the priestess.

Queen of Heaven

Before we move on, let's just explore the term Queen of Heaven, so we get a really full picture of the goddess inhabiting these temples. The term derives from the Old Testament and appears twice in the Book of Jeremiah. We hear that the women were "kneading and baking bread for the Queen of Heaven" in Jeremiah 7:18.

I think it's fair to say that Jeremiah is not a fan, because in 44:17-25 we hear how he pleads with the Israelites to cease honouring this goddess because the Lord had become angry at their disobedience and idolatry and was likely to punish them with calamity. He implores them that God has spoken to him and threatened that worse punishments lie in wait.

But the people refuse.

They say they are going to continue pouring libations to the goddess, and even go as far as to credit her with the grace they used to enjoy at God's mercy.

There is an inference that the Queen of Heaven existed as a consort to Yahweh and that it was she who was the source of his favour.

But who was she?

Well, in this guise, it's fairly certain she was Ashtoreth, wife of Ba'al, but the term can encompass any of the incarnations of The Goddess of Mesopotamia or the Near East. So, we can consider that she is also Asherah, Astarte, Inanna, Anat, Ishtar, Isis, Nut, Neith, Hera or Juno.

Where Astarte was the Hellenised version of the Middle Eastern Goddess, Ashtoreth and Ishtar were her Semitic counterparts. Ishtar was the Assyrian, Babylonian and Akkadian goddess of love, sex, fertility, and war. Believed to be the daughter of the supreme ruler of the Sumerian pantheon, the sky god Anu. Ishtar was depicted by a star with either 6, 8 or 18 rays inhabiting a circle. The sign incarnated her as the planet Venus and sometimes she is depicted wearing what seems to be the familiar "bee" skirt.

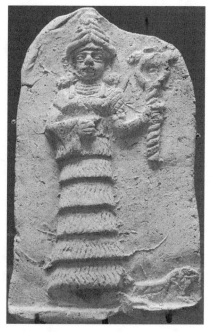

The Babylonian goddess Ishtar wearing the "bee" skirt. Early second millennium BCE. Louvre. Photograph by Marie-Lan Nguyen.

Her story has many parallels with Inanna's, but also now brings in a much stronger agricultural bias too. The story goes that

Ishtar decided she must go to the underworld. As she passed through each of the gates, she had to remove another item of clothing, until in a total state of undress, she faced Ereshkigal, who, by return, in her fury threw 60 diseases at her and retained her in the underworld.

Absent from the upperworld, there was no power of fertility, so the sterile world began to fade. All fertility left the Earth.

Eventually the god Ea had to intervene, liberated her, and she returned back, through the gates, recovering her clothes.

On her return, she asks Gilgamesh to make her his wife, but he declines. Furious, she goes to see Anu, and demands to be given the Bull of the Heavens, which she then sets upon Gilgamesh and his ally, Enkidu. Enkidu rails against the goddess, insulting her and he has to be put to death.

Dates, wool, meat, and grain all came under her dominion, and she is often referred to lovingly as "Lady of the Date Clusters". An early representation of Ishtar was incarnated as the very grain storehouse, and her symbol came to be the grain store gates.

Her formidable firepower seems to derive from another myth where she commands thunderstorms and rain. Commonly, she, like Aphrodite, was considered to be the protectress of prostitutes and she too is often associated with sacred prostitution.

Until around the time of the Second World War, the stories about Corinth, Eryx and other tales connected to the Syrian Goddess were generally accepted as strange, rather unsavoury, but fact.

Scholastic niggles were definitely audible, but no-one could really get a handle on what exactly was wrong, or indeed, if it *was* wrong, where the crossroads had become obscured.

Today, opinion seems unanimous that sacred prostitution, apart from being a rather vulgar title, discredits the agency of the priestess. Sacred sex need not imply prostitution. In considering Aphrodite's role as goddess of love and sex, for example, any sexual ritual to her would be deemed pure.

To her, all sex is sacred.

Changes in perception have been gradual, requiring concerted efforts to unpick the narratives of two thousand years, but it now seems widely agreed that the stories were sabotaged by the writers of the Hebrew Bible, aided and abetted by early Christian writers and travel commentators like Herodotus.

Wait. What?

Herodotus is a bad guy? That's a bitter pill to swallow!

It had completely passed me by that the Father of History is also known in some quarters as the Father of Lies.

I will concede, though, that I, too, had been rather incredulous of his intrepid adventures on the seas, travelling thousands of miles, spending long periods of time with the natives, documenting strange and marvellous facts. I can remember being amazed, when I was writing the Cannabis Medicine book, that the gods had been astonishingly generous in ensuring a Scythian funeral took place, replete with hallucinogens concocted with an oversized cauldron-bong, right in front of his eyes at the very moment he was in the right place... the perfect content for his book... but still my perception was not shaken.

But now, it seems, general consensus is that it's unlikely Herodotus could be just one man (especially without the speed of air travel), but perhaps a team of many, and like any commentator's work, it can be difficult to read their texts without perceiving bias, in this case, a moralistic early Christian bias.

So, when we read about the "wholly shameful" custom by which every woman "once in her life" had intercourse near the temple of Aphrodite (Ishtar) with the first stranger who threw "a silver coin" into her lap, we might start to feel a little uneasy about the association between the priestess Melissa and the worship of the goddess. Herodotus implies the priestess' actions of ritual sex were nothing extraordinary and indeed every woman was expected to worship this way. He writes:

> *Every woman born in the country must once in her life go and sit down in the precinct of Venus and there have sex with a stranger. Many of the wealthier sort, who are too proud to mix with the others, drive in covered carriages to the precinct, followed by a goodly train of attendants, and there take their station. But the larger number seat themselves in the holy enclosure with wreaths of string about their heads... and the strangers pass along them to make their choice.*
>
> *A woman who has taken her seat is not allowed to come home till one of the strangers throws a silver coin into her lap and takes him with her beyond the holy ground. When he throws the coin, he says these words: "The Goddess Mylitta prosper thee." (Venus is called Mylitta by the Assyrians.) The silver coin may be any size; it cannot be refused, for that is forbidden by law, since once it is thrown it is sacred. The woman goes with the first man who throws her money and rejects no-one. When she has gone with him, and so satisfied The Goddess, she returns home, and from that time forth no gift however great will prevail with her. Such of the women who are tall and beautiful are soon released, but others who are ugly have to stay a long time before they can fulfil the law. Some have waited three or four years in the precinct.*

In *De Deo Syria*, Lucian also asserts that women who refused to shave their heads in mourning for Adonis' passing, risked judgement in sacred law: "For a single day they [had to] stand offering their beauty for sale... [in a] market... open to foreigners only, and the payment [became] an offering to Aphrodite [Astarte]."

In 1941, historian Beatrice Brooks voiced her concern about this anomaly suggesting an "improbable percentage of the population [of Mesopotamia and Syria-Canaan] must have been either secular or religious prostitutes of some sort." I see her point. It does seem we are reading sensationalist headlines designed to make us look. But how much evidence is there for it?

In 1928, a peasant farmer, ploughing his field, came upon a cave and opened it, revealing a tomb. The necropolis, located near to the modern seaport of Minet el-Beida, in modern-day Syria, was later revealed to be part of the vast temple complex of Ugarit, believed to have been destroyed during the fall of the Bronze Age in 1200 BCE.

The site was worked for over 40 years by archaeologist Claude Schaeffer from the Musée Archeologique in Strasbourg, with just a small break from 1940-47. The finds, including 150 clay tablets, found at various points during the excavation, vastly overhauled our understanding of Canaanite life and gave detailed insights into their worship of Ba'al and his divine wife, Asherah.

In her paper, "Priestesses and 'Sacred Prostitutes' in the ancient Near East", Johanna Stuckey of the University of York describes in detail the suspected plotters in the vilification of The Goddess.

Her first piece of evidence is strong and literally made me gasp aloud at the double standards still rife today when I read the entry under "prostitute" from Webster's Dictionary:

> ... a woman who engages in sexual intercourse for money; whore; harlot.

second,

> ... a man who engages in sexual acts for money.

She explains that, until recently, scholars had not distinguished between a woman as a prostitute and a woman who engaged in sacred sex, reminding us that sexual pleasure in a ritual setting does not necessarily imply prostitution.

The word *qᵉdeshah* is mentioned in just four places in the Old Testament, mostly in the sections between Deuteronomy and 2 Kings which talk about the new Israelite community. In all cases, the word is translated into the English version as "sacred prostitute", and whilst texts from Ugarit refer to their high priests and priestesses as *qdsham* – it is recognised here as meaning "consecrated ones." Ugarit offers no evidence of sexual roles or indeed that sacred "prostitution" played a part there at all.

The Mesopotamian word *quadashitu*, which is associated with female cultic personnel, had been taken to read as prostitute, however, we now understand it to mean "Holy or set apart woman", or perhaps "anointed one".

Chapter 13

Raising Brood

In Greece, April is considered sacred to Aphrodite. I love the gorgeous symbolism of how beauty and sexuality return to the Earth. With that resurgence of growth, so too does life inside the hive.

As I write, today's temperature is 15 degrees Celsius and tomorrow, it's predicted to soar to 21 degrees. There was plenty of activity at the local hives as I walked across the fields this morning. Bees popping in and out. The odd one or two heading off on longer journeys. Daffodils bobbed their heads in the breeze and every few minutes or so, another insect emerged from a golden trumpet.

Foragers industriously scouted pollen and I hoped one that zoomed disconcertingly close to my ear might head off to suss out my own springtime flowers.

Just as fast as bees emerged, others buzzed back in, the baskets on the backs of their legs laden with gold. I puzzled, for a few moments, if fewer flowers in spring and smaller hive populations could be a coincidental correlation, then instantly chastised myself, because certainly, nothing about bees happens by chance.

Inside the hive, I sensed workers busily constructing more comb and the queen methodically laying egg after egg to fill it, fertilising most to generate yet more workers and laying the odd unfertilised ones to make drones. I imagined her carefully standing astride each cell calculating how much room she had for each. Throughout spring and summer, as the colony rapidly evolves, she will lay up to 2000 eggs a day, ready to take advantage of the explosion of colour that is just a few short weeks away.

The queen doesn't eat the same pollen and nectar as the other bees. She doesn't have time, and she needs far more nutrition. To allow her to focus on her important role, her attendants, imagined in the myths as *The Charites* or *Three Graces*, groom and feed her with food they have predigested, processing proteins into amino acids which she speedily metabolises into fuel to produce more eggs.

Each day, she lays so many that they exceed her total body weight.

The beekeeper will soon have decisions to make, and it's likely he will separate the hive, placing in a new section – a queen excluder – to isolate her from the rest of the hive so there is comb that she can no longer get to. This leaves the majority of the cells free for the bees to fill with honey; delicious sweetness to feed the hive and, of course, the beekeeper's family too.

The balance of how much honey the keeper takes forms a sacred contract between his intuition and the bees. The more they make, the better reserves they have for winter. The more the keeper takes, the harder it becomes for the bees, so many modern keepers supplement by feeding them sugar syrup and fondant to sustain them in the cold. Many things account for the difference between bee guardian or keeper, but most assuredly, this one is key.

Developing good intuition is key to any animal husbandry but is particularly so for bees. A healthy hive depends on the keeper maintaining keen observations of the delicate balance between the queen making plenty of brood cells and knowing when the hive is ready to swarm.

She secretes that pheromone known as QMP, or Queen Mandibular Pheromone. Its chemical signature means, "The queen is in residence. No need to make more queens." Her attendants reek of it after feeding her, and they spread it around the hive. As long as there is QMP circulating, workers' ovaries are deactivated, rendering them sterile.

Should the unthinkable happen, and the colony loses its queen, it faces a cascade of innumerable changes and challenges. If the queen's scent is absent for more than 30 minutes, pheromone signalling alters. Workers' ovaries begin to produce eggs and they too begin to lay, but having never had nuptial flights, they've no sperm stores to fertilise them. Thus, it might be that hundreds of bees are happily flying in and out with pollen, furiously making honey to feed the growing brood, but the parthenogenic births will eventually, of course, lead to the colony's demise, with no females to do any of the work or continue the line. This phenomenon is called *"Laying Workers"*.

Concurrently then, workers speedily begin protocols of raising queen cells, in the hopes of making the hive *"Queenright"*. Nurse bees identify which "normal" cells to make into princesses and begin gorging them on royal jelly. In addition, the keeper might want to take control of the situation himself and *"Requeen"* by introducing a queen from another hive or supplier.

An absentee queen isn't the only reason the colony might raise new princesses though.

Most often, it's that the hive has become too cramped, so the colony wants more space to continue growing its family. Bees are entirely ruled by urges. The drive to build is irresistible, but each bee is subject to a much larger plan. It's the colony (rather than the individual bee) that is the animal, and the animal needs to reproduce. Queen cells may be a sign of a hive getting ready to divide into two colonies – that is to swarm. Many keepers split their hive as a means of colony contraception, placing some of the frames into a new hive so the bees imagine they have already swarmed and upgraded to a bigger home with more room to grow. Hopefully, this should now mean they remain happily in their hives, but as bee mentors repeatedly like to tell me, we should remember that bees don't tend to read the books!

Monitoring the reproductive cycle requires a keen eye, looking out for much larger acorn-shaped queen cells, stretched out and polished, ready to hatch.

If a split doesn't take place, the colony will swarm, which for many guardians, as for the bees, is a blissfully happy occasion – as long as you don't lose your bees!

They may also be made for *supersedure*, if the queen is not laying well enough, or she is ailing in some way. Potentially her pheromones are fading, so she can't be smelt as strongly as she was. The workers secure the colony's future by **superseding** the queen to support her by raising a secondary queen. Sometimes, the queen happily accepts the supersedure and will move around the hive, quite contentedly with one of her daughters, both laying eggs. More often than not though, the two queens will fight and always to the death.

Chapter 14

The Blood Mysteries

We'll leave book learning and Knowledge Lectures behind from here on in. These reflections of the womb shamans have been brought down entirely from meditating and dreaming with Lemon Balm plant, with Melissa essential oil, CO_2, and hydrolat, from using meditation techniques I have learnt and, of course, from spending time with the actual insects.

In itself, that presents myriad opportunities and just as many pitfalls. The major difficulty is information gained in this way is never linear. Sometimes it is sparked by something I've read. I've asked the hive, then dreamed on it. Then some other symbolism or place has come through and I've headed off to grok that. Compound that with the many interpretations of women in the hive consciousness, who have added to the Mysteries for over five thousand years, well as you can imagine, it can all get a little jumbled.

M. officinalis, the plant, is profoundly involved with gynaecology, reducing period pain, balancing mood, and even guarding against post-natal depression. Since the priestesses were Melissae and connected with a plant that protects women's sexual and reproductive health, I wanted to see if I could find that. People had been searching for the secrets of the Eleusinian Mysteries for eons. So had I and I'd grown bored of it. This seemed far more interesting to find. Could the Lemon Balm plant be the keeper of the Blood Mysteries, I conjectured? So, what I decided I wanted the priestesses to help me find, wasn't the Mysteries themselves, I wanted them to show me their sexual medicine.

Maybe, I shouldn't have been surprised that it would take me on a journey of family planning and colony control. Nevertheless, despite the plant's primary use being for emotional stability or gynaecological issues, discovering that the Aphrodite medicine would take me on the same journey, took me entirely by surprise.

It's a tale of preparation and planning, and sometimes emergency measures. How to separate the queen and her brood in cases of illness, accidents, or other critical measures. And if it's done right, it's the tale of wealth, beauty, and romance.

Most of all, it's the legacy of a lifetime of honey.

It's not taught, as far as I know, as part of priestess training, nevertheless as a plant healer I've found it perhaps the most fascinating to explore.

I wanted to know if a Melissa association with menstruation could be found in the myths.

I'll save you the frustration I endured.

It's not there.

Nowhere.

I don't know why I expected it would be, because surely, it was carefully folded into the Red Tent canvas.

Eventually, it would be a piece of work a ghostwriting customer had asked me to consult on that moved my thoughts. I realised I had overlooked something that's supposed to be my specialty, and yet distracted as I was by bees, it had been hidden in plain sight.

Meridians.

I was so annoyed at myself for not having considered it before.

Aphrodite's girdle!

Aphrodite's girdle appears in the fifth *Homeric Hymn* where Hera tries to manipulate the goddess of love into giving her some of her skills of seduction to trick Zeus. The girdle was imbued with the power to fuel anyone with desire.

The earliest acupuncture and bee venom therapy was known to have originated in China and ancient Greece.[60] The girdle is the sexual and gynaecological meridian!

Ancient Greek acupuncture practice is outlined in the 11th chapter of Hippocrates' book *On Human Nature*. It is also spoken of by Pliny and Galen. Originally acupuncture wasn't done with needles but with beestings placed at strategic places along the meridians.

Greek acupuncturist, Alexandros Tilikidis, relates Hippocrates' explanation is designed similarly to the Chinese modality, operating on a meridian system primarily consisting of four pairs of channels. Just as in Traditional Chinese Medicine (TCM), points are located along this channel system. Bees were placed along the meridians and encouraged to sting to create immune responses and bring physiological processing into balance. Hippocrates names this as "his blood-letting therapeutic technique" (whether he also used leeches on the points, is unclear).

The girdle meridian (sometimes called the belt) sits across the top of the hips where the base of the corset sits and is the only meridian line that runs horizontally across the body. Its Chinese name is Dai Mai or Belt Vessel.

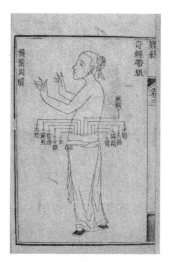

Belt Vessel (Dai Mai), Chinese woodcut, 1817 edition of Bian Que maishu nan jing.

Originating in the kidney meridian, it moves essence (what the Chinese call *jing*), through the body, then generates *qi* or in the closest ancient Greek representation, vital breath or pneuma.

Along with *qi* (energy/function) and *shen* (spirit or spirits), jing completes the Three Treasures. It is stored in the kidneys, governs growth, development, and reproduction, and holds the body's energy reserves. When jing is depleted, physical changes take place especially within the sexual body.

Libido and fertility rely entirely on jing balance. If jing is deficient, so will libido be; the ability to conceive, maintain an erection or to ejaculate are all compromised. The girdle meridian is the primary way to balance this.

I imagined the priestess moving the energies just as Chinese practitioners have done for thousands of years. The manifestation of jing moves through each of the changing elements to warm, to move, defend, contain, and transform. There is a sense of warming the blood from the yang kidney, then cooling it as it passes through yin. For those unfamiliar with TCM, the movement of energy through the elements is depicted as a five-pointed star – the same sign that shows the retrogrades of Venus and indeed of sorceresses themselves. It's a pentacle.

The meridian is used mainly to help heal bladder and yeast infections and STIs, but is also extremely useful to loosen the hips in labour to give the baby's head more room to pass through.

As 21st century beings, we pathologically lean towards a yang kidney disposition. Call it the patriarchal body if you like... so much yang... so much competitive nature, aggression...

That lack of balance manifests as insomnia, fitful tempers, poor memory, stress...

Every other meridian runs vertically up and down the body, so this one, running through it, binds all the others, holding them in balance. It harmonises the hips, waist, and legs, and influences the lower *jaio* responsible for problems in the pelvic area and to the legs and lower back. Clinical presentations range from chronic lower back pain, STDs, yeast infections, joint pain/ inflammation and chronic or acute UTIs.

Other telling signs can be urinary burning, itching and soreness.

It harmonises the liver and gall bladder meridians so if it's out of balance, then there will be insufficient power to fuel *agni*. Metabolism struggles to bring enough warmth to transform nutrients which presents as loose stools, diarrhoea, bloating, and other signs of digestive weakness. Likewise, it balances stools, guarding against straining and alleviating pressure on haemorrhoids. It is said to balance excess belly fat.

Clearly, if agni is weak, and there is not enough internal fire to fuel metabolism, this will have similar repercussions for sexuality, which means bad news in terms of both libido and fertility. Conception and pregnancy are very much guided and controlled by jing. They believe it to be stored in the kidneys, and if there is a deficiency in this area, this also shows itself as jing weakness. Physically this presents as infertility or repeated miscarriage.

It dries dampness in UTIs and yeast infections, as well as regulating external genitalia issues such as Bartholin's cysts. The girdle meridian mediates gynaecological functions such as irregular periods, pelvic inflammatory disease, and miscarriage.

Jing governs the material basis of the body, so: the blood, tissues, bones, and teeth. It is predominately yin, energetically, and thus pertains to the feminine nature. Anything yin is cooling, nourishing, and drying. It is said a person is born with a fixed amount of jing, but then from the moment of birth, its reservoir begins to deplete. Daily stress, illness, substance abuse, and sexual challenges all steal its energy. The biggest physical strains on jing are sperm production, menstrual blood, and pregnancy. It's impossible, of course, to ever recapture the levels we are born with, but with care it can be bolstered and preserved. It is nourished, postnatally by food, exercise, study, and by spiritual work.

If we imagine the ribbons of the corset, running down the back, the girdle closes on the point known as Sea of Ming Men, or The Gate of Life. Brisk or light, circular rubbing over this point helps balance the system and gentle passage across the girdle meridian can be a blissful help against pubic symphysis pain during pregnancy.

Why I'd not thought of it before is beyond me, because I'd been seeing these endless loops of fighting going on, over the girdle, in dreams.

I'd know it was Aphrodite's girdle, but then watch as Hercules stole it from the Amazonian Queen, Hippolyta, then I'd see Adonis being killed by a boar which Artemis would claim as hers in retaliation to Aphrodite cursing and killing her devotee Hippolytus, who in turn was Theseus' son, born after Theseus had raped said Hippolyta. "Yes," said Theseus then, soberly. "This is *synoikismos*." (Synoikismos means something akin to "Bringing together".)

All of these girdle things do happen in the myths, and I knew what my brain was reminding me now. The girdle meridian also regulates hip and waist pain and sciatica. Hippolytus... *-itis* means inflammation. Inflammation of the hips.

It *might* be a coincidence, but it's a hell of a one if it is.

The Bee Mistress most assuredly is The Queen of Synchronicity.

You would also be careful of overstimulating this band of points in massage, since it has the power to unlock memories connected to sexual trauma such as abuse and rape.

If the girdle marks the bottom of the corset, now we start to see the midline stitching, and indeed the line that could be construed as creating the chastity belt.

The conception vessel (Chinese name Ren Mai) originates from the kidney. From there, it runs down the back, comes up between the legs, over the perineum (the point known as Ren 1), then up the front midline, to just under the middle of the bottom lip of the mouth.

Imagine the suggestive finger gently tracing up the chest, to lift the chin.

Its energy flows right through the main focal areas of Melissa work. In dream work, for example, the energy is dropped down into what's called the womb space. This could be the womb, but likewise it might also be accessed by a man, or indeed a woman who has had a hysterectomy.

The conception vessel marks the section where sacral chakra energy moves up to the heart chakra and is fundamental to the energetic interchange between the uterus and blood.

To be clear, as previously stated, the Western energy centres used in Bee Shamanism do not have exact correlations to the more commonly known Eastern ones, however, after much internal wrangling, I've decided to leave the names, positions, and applications of these necktary centres in oral tradition where they belong. Suffice it to say, most of the centres correlate to the same pathway as the conception vessel, which by extension governs the female gynaecological life. It affects puberty, menstruation, fertility, pregnancy, childbirth, postpartum healing, perimenopause, and menopause.

Both the girdle and conception meridians are what are known as Extraordinary Vessels. They offer additional knowledge and healing to the ordinary eight meridians. Like all other extraordinary vessels, the conception vessel is a vast energetic well that the other meridians can draw upon if they become depleted. Thus, this is a wonderful access point for things like scanty or absent periods, to bring the body back into balance after childbirth or miscarriage, or indeed if there is a natural weakening of yang in menopause.

The conception vessel does more than just nourish. It actively moves energy through the uterus and supplementary organs that inhabit the pelvic cavity which include the bladder and, for men, the prostate too. These points can be used for any number of symptoms including chronic bladder problems, fibroids, abdominal masses, ovarian cysts, hernias, or prostate issues.

The conception vessel can be accessed via the kidney meridian (which has Aphrodite's water energy) and through the respiratory tools of the lung meridian. (That's Artemis' realm.) It connects to both. It helps descent lung qi (when that's not happening, you get coughing and wheezing), as well as helping the kidneys to grasp qi.

Taken together, this means that Ren Mai helps with respiration, aiding both in- and exhalation. As such, it is frequently used to treat asthma. This breath of life seems related to pneuma.

Similarly Greek medics believed a person to have a designated reservoir of pneuma, that is to say: "Breath of God", a person's vital spirit, soul, or creative force.

According to Rufus of Ephesus, a writer from the first century CE, pneuma had a medical component of being air, which passed through the lungs, but it was also construed as air in motion, or indeed something vital to life. Certain things, they believed, including sexual activity, depleted this.

Perhaps the most famous representation of pneuma was the spirited smoke drawn up into the oracle's vagina. The pneuma kisses the first point of the conception vessel meridian, point Ren 1, the perineum, to the lay men and women.

Found midway between the anus and scrotum in men, and between the labia and the anus in women, Ren 1 alleviates impotence, improves seminal emission, remedies genital pain, and nourishes pneuma or spirit.

It may be surplus to requirement to explain what the kidney and bladder meridians do but suffice it to say the kidney meridian marks the front of the corset. It traces the top neckline and the front panels, where the bladder marks the edges of the lacing panel at the back.

After understanding what Aphrodite's influence might be on sexuality, I was intrigued to know how the Greeks might have viewed menstruation, given that this is such a vital part of the Lemon Balm medicine, accepting that it is all probably from a male perspective since there are so few women's thoughts written down.

Interestingly, many of their ideas about sexuality are expressed as heat, or in the case of menstruation, an absence of it. It's satisfying to see the archetypes speaking in their medicine, Mars being the hot aggressive divine masculine, against the cooling nature of Venus.

Menstruation

Hesiod is our first written evidence of this correlation of heat and ardour from the eighth century BCE. The idea was probably not originally his but more likely already circulating in traditional folk medicine of the time. He described how heat appeared to compromise men's performance, impeding semen from being drawn from its sources, which were, he said, in the head and knee.

I was quizzical about why sperm would be stored in a man's patella, found no particular explanations, and I now find someone proposing properly even more delightful. What it *did* make me think, though, is flower semen is collected on bees faces and on the back of their knees! I'm not sure if that's a weird coincidence or not...

He further explains heat seems not to affect women in the same way, because their bodies are too cold and clammy to produce semen thus, they menstruate instead, producing their own marvellous life-giving fluids. Sunshine, though, he implied, made women rampant. *"In the draining heat, when goats are plumpest and wine is finest, and women are on heat, but men are weak..."*

It sounds rather foolish when we lay it out like that, but actually, Hippocrates and Galen both taught similar doctrine in their work with the humours and it does, of course, in turn echo the Chinese Medicine of *jing* I have laid out.

Here we see the first tension between Venus and Mars. Mars is blood, unable to stay away.

When menstruation first began at puberty the parthenos donned a girdle to mark the occasion.

Screwed up cloths were used as tampons. The verb "to tamp" means to plug a hole. Obviously, Tampax completely usurped the context.

The girdle was fixed using a special knot, that the betrothed would untie, but only after asking permission from Artemis. The girdle was later offered to Artemis after the maiden had had her first sexual experience (which may or may not have taken place on the wedding night, of course!). Artemis thus gained the epithet: "Lysizones", "releaser of the girdle".[19]

Artemis then also untied the girdle, one last time, when the soon to be new mother felt her first labour pains.

Soranus of Ephesus was a gynaecologist who wrote a four-volume treatise about women's medicine. Precious little is known about his life except that he was already dead by the time Galen began writing in c. 180 BCE. Seemingly sympathetic to the moans and groans of menstruation, Soranus described symptoms of lethargy, muscle aching, sluggishness, excessive nausea, hot flushes, and loss of appetite. He advises that each woman should do what she feels is best for her during her period whether that be to rest or just participate in very light activities.

He rejects the idea of menstruation being a healthy purgative completely, arguing that its objective was solely to facilitate conception. Thus, women approaching menopause should take care to ensure their menses faded away slowly and had a moral obligation to take all actions necessary to try to prolong the bleeding as long as possible.

He recommends using suppositories or injections to do this but does not elucidate which herbs he'd prescribe.

The ancient word for the female external genitalia is *choiros*.

The word was used to either describe the genitals of little girls or to older women's parts if they were depilated. (How does that come up in polite conversation...?)

The word *choiros* has an interesting linguistic dimension, in that if it is used in the masculine it means "female genitalia" but in the feminine, it's "pig". Thus, your choiros was your piggy, and presumably, if you were a harlot who advertised, yours would be smooth, depilated with beeswax presumably.

Aristophanes, always guaranteed to put a smutty slant on things, refers to menstrual cloths as "pig pens".

In *Lysistrata*, he jests that the men look like they are wearing "pig-pens" (choirokomeion) round their thighs.

So, is the joke here about wearing something around your piggy that looks quite bulky – such as a home-made menstrual pad?

Nope. The stage direction in the libretto betrays that when they open their cloaks, it's a rather cheeky line of erect penises that steals the show.

Hesiod warned that men should never wash in water that women had already used in case they were somehow polluted by menstrual blood. Presumably then, women were encouraged to bathe during their periods.

Dioscorides cites no less than 100 herbs and concoctions that can start a period, Pliny the Elder cites 90. The "fumigation" was considered to be a vital cure-all for women, because whilst their identity was firmly placed in the womb, the uterus was believed to be prone to go wandering freely around the body placing excess pressure on other organs. If the womb was not in the right position, how could a woman conceive?

Thus, if she missed a period, blood, it was thought, could pool in the uterus causing health issues and the womb to wander.

The fumigation was a rigorous process. Herbs and water were placed into an amphora, then buried in the ground. The neck of the jug tightly sealed with a reed leading up into the womb. It was a long slow and potentially uncomfortable process. In Egypt, similar practices took place, smoking with resins rather than herbal steams.

I find it fascinating that many of the spells in the Graeco-Egyptian magical papyri begin with the words "fumigation with herbs". Perhaps a reference to how much more potently a woman's sexual energy was viewed, than today. Her power was magnified manifold as her sexual fluids dripped back onto the earth.

Pliny has many thoughts about menstruation. Some rational, others… not so much.

Having a period in a lunar or solar eclipse bode very poorly for a woman or indeed any man who had sex with her during it, apparently. Any man who had suicidal thoughts, and then had sex with a menstruating woman would surely go on to kill himself.

Incidentally, all these are taken from *In Bed With The Greeks* by Paul Chrystal. Some are delightfully funny, but this one stuck. Pliny says:

…it is one of the first rules that people must wash themselves clean before they take the honey, also bees hate scurf, and women's menstruation.

I'm fascinated by this, and oddly about three days after I wrote this last paragraph, someone asked the exact question in a women beekeepers' Facebook page. Do bees know if you're menstruating? Overwhelmingly, the women agreed, yes, their bees did know, and they didn't like it if they went near the hive when they were bleeding.

Did that inform Melissae beekeeping? To avoid the dark of the moon and perhaps spend more time with the bees when it was full. I'm the wrong person to ask if they are different. I'm too chicken to open the hive at night.

Contraception

I'm inquisitive as to whether there is significance in there being so little written about contraception in the age. Perhaps women thought it had naught to do with men and kept it hidden within the confines of Thesmophoria. Bee shamanism teachings about the priestess being able to control when the sperm meets the egg suggests that may be so.

I find it interesting that Thesmophoria, Demeter's most important festival, took place between the 11th-13th of the month. Months opened with the new moon, so if we are to believe that each woman bled during the lunar darkness, the ritual took place under the waxing beauty, just as the female community was preparing to ovulate. The sheer power of that connotation is astonishing. All women ovulating together, the joint fertility of the polis.

On the second day of the ritual, they are said to have sat on the leaves of the lygos tree, *Vitex agnus castus*. Its leaves make wonderfully fertile medicines that modulate levels of oestrogen and progesterone to aid conception.

That the women quietly sat on them suggests to me an unspoken agreement that these are the days to be chaste if you, like Gaia, have had enough of being pregnant. Perhaps this is the herbal equivalent of "hacking off his rutting phallus".

The Hippocratic corpus recommends drinking *Misy*, a solution of dilute copper sulphate, as a contraceptive. You may recall the priestess of Aphrodite controlled sales and transactions of copper.[61] Misy is also the Greek name for the island of Crete.[62]

Soranus had another engaging notion. He prescribes water that a blacksmith has used to cool iron.

Bizarrely in the context of the text, the Egyptian Kahun Papyrus recommends using crocodile faeces either as contraceptive or as abortifacient. I have no idea how those were taken and neither do I think I want to know.

First catch your crocodile...

Please do not house said croc on your tits. One breast may become jealous and then you'll have to farm another.

Do you remember the Maenads? The women of Dionysos cult?

If the Maenads are the darker side of the Melissae, or maybe somehow their shadow, one would suspect they may have something to do with disrupting nature, would you agree?

I keep thinking about their staff, their thyrsus...

A fennel stalk topped with a fir cone and twisted round with ivy.

Fennel is phyto estrogenic, modulating the flow of oestrogen, too.

The favoured Greek abortifacient agent is believed to have been a plant called silphium, and while the exact species of the plant is unknown, it is thought to have been some kind of giant fennel, possibly also depicted on a Minoan seal.[61] Those thyrsus staffs are very long. It's not beyond the realms of possibility that the fennel was giant.

Bathing

Anyone who has spent any time watching bees will likely smile at how Aphrodite was so often depicted bathing. There is something so human-like about how bees groom themselves. It was this behaviour that first made me fall in love with them.

In honeys, these are the water bees, of course, just like the nurse bees who had cared for Zeus, but for me, the original relationship was first forged with big fat hairy bumbles.

I'm not a boastful person, but what I will say, is our paddling pool is feckin' awesome. About 5ft square, complete with its own seats and cup holders, I am a big fan. As a Cancerian, perhaps it's not surprising I would have an intimate relationship with water, but it jars with me how much it uses up. So, each night after dinner, I head off to pour a few watering cans of its contents over the roses, on a three-day loop. Fill it up, enjoy it clean for a day and a half then, when the third day comes, all the chlorine has evaporated and I can put some in the pond to look after my beloved newts.

The binding ritual fills me with joy, not least because bumblebees often need rescuing from it, meaning I selfishly delight in the honour of them wanting to sit with me for a while. We lose the odd one, but I've developed a rather keen eye for the striped guys since most seem to go swimming about 3pm. The water sparkles against the clean white base and they just cannot wait to dive in. Some days I can have as many as four rescuees sitting on my hand, happily preening, and drying themselves after their baths.

Rather than women who seem to be like bees, these insects almost transform, as if minuscule hairy ladies.

Only today, one sat with me for a good 20 minutes, first sitting to catch her breath then very carefully drying herself and combing her hair. Clearly aware of their importance in her pollen quest, she carefully washed her face, unfurled the hairs on her legs, then spent time languorously rubbing her bum dry with her "hands". Every now and then she'd assess whether her wings were dry yet, almost as if she was buzzing me thanks as she went. I lay prostrate on the decking, wrapped my fingers round a deep blue salvia being greedily nuzzled by a gang of carder bees, hoping to coax her onto the flower. But not until the very last hair was back to being soft and fuzzy, did she finally agree to leave my hand and buzz off to land on a rose.

It was a blissful few moments spent.

As an aromatherapist, it's always been very clear to me that the urge to look youthful far outweighs the desire to stay healthy for most people. It's easy to see how the goddess of beauty could inspire such a following. Wax, honey, royal jelly; they all have uses in a beauty parlour.

About five years ago, I had the good fortune to visit the Roman spas in Bath, where another water goddess had been honoured by the name of Sulis Minerva. In one of the areas, amongst the ruined walls and pillars, was an enormous video projection. The haunting film transfixed me. There, I was reunited with my co-workers from two thousand years before. Ghostly masseuses with elegant dresses and prettily-styled hair floated before me, reverently mixing healing oils. Clients lay on softly draped couches, luxuriating in repose. Elixirs were poured like libations from terracotta jugs, then skilfully worked into the skin. Hairdressers, beauticians, and therapists all working tirelessly amidst the mineral steam.

I found the exhibit electrifying. It saddened me that some areas of the museum were so crammed that we lost the children in body crushes, yet I watched the women ply their trade in solitude, quite speechless at how ethereally the designers had managed to transport me through time. The women though, key workers in this majestic space, seemed no longer of interest to the crowds.

To find that Corinth had also been a spa town thrilled me. A prosperous town, Acrocorinth as it was then called, formed the strategic trading link from the east of Greece to its west coast, Athens, and was always teeming with sailors and merchants. Perhaps most famous of its associations was its temple to Aphrodite, complete with 1000 prostitutes, its hetaerae (courtesans) enjoyed a similar reputation as the Melissae of

Eryx. Acrocorinth was a place of partying and loose morals, but in the home of Aphrodisia, one of Greece's most spectacular festivals, where The Goddess was taken down to the water to be ritually washed, bathing also played an enormous part.

Public bathing, spas, beauty, and wealth all bubbling up in Corinth.

Archaeologist Jane Biers describes how excavations have uncovered multiple Roman bathhouses in Corinth. Certainly nine, probably 10, maybe as many as 11 buildings were constructed to house one of the greatest pastimes of the Roman age, bathing. Pausanias described visiting one as he'd travelled north along the Lechaion Road. Biers and her team had been able to identify the very one he had spoken of, making it the earliest of the ones they had studied, dating it at around the second century CE. It's a little later than the Greek priestesses, heading into Roman, but she reports evidence circulating of bathing taking place here much earlier.

The title of her paper, "Lavari est Vivere", delights me. Taken from graffiti found in the area it speaks of how the baths are ultimately one of the things that make Corinthian life worth living. Public bathing was not just about cleanliness and health, but more, it was a place to meet friends and make new contacts, a place to flaunt affluence or look jealously on.

A place to bathe, to have your hair plucked or coiffed, for a facial or massage, the bathhouse was the networking hub of antiquity.

Aphrodite was the patron Goddess at Acrocorinth and had three shrines dedicated to her. As formerly mentioned, this was the famous temple of the courtesans.

Strabo describes it:

The temple of Aphrodite [in Korinthos in the days of the tyrant Kypselos] was so rich that it owned more than a thousand temple slaves, courtesans, whom both men and women had dedicated to The Goddess. And therefore, it was also on account of these women that the city was crowded with people and grew rich; for instance, the ship captains freely squandered their money, and hence the proverb, "Not for every man is the voyage to Korinthos." ... Now the summit [of the Akrokorinthos] has a small temple of Aphrodite; and below the summit is the spring Peirene... At any rate, Euripides says, "I am come, having left Akrokorinthos that is washed on all sides, the sacred hill-city of Aphrodite." [...] Korinthos, there, on account of the multitude of courtesans, who were sacred to Aphrodite, outsiders resorted in great numbers and kept holiday. And the merchants and soldiers who went there squandered all their money so that the following proverb arose in reference to them: "Not for every man is the voyage to Korinthos."

He sells the hill short. The tiny sanctuary requires a climb of no less than 1700ft.

Prostitution

The beautifully coiffed and educated hetaerae could apparently charge up to a thousand drachma a night, which was then turned over to the temple. But the hetera Melissa priestess was top rung, prime rump, and set aside for the elite. Presumably, those who could afford her were few and far between.

On the bottom rung of the ladder, with skirt hems filthy from the gutter, were the *pornai*. Far from being mistresses of their hives, these poor souls were subject to the whims of their pimps and madams. Protecting their assets, the bosses came up with an ingenious marketing tool to help them scout for trade.

Excavations have uncovered specially made sandals that left messages as they walked. The footprint imprint reads: "ΑΚΟΛΟΥΘΕΙ AKOLOUTHEI"[63] (*Fig. 14b*) – "Follow me".[63]

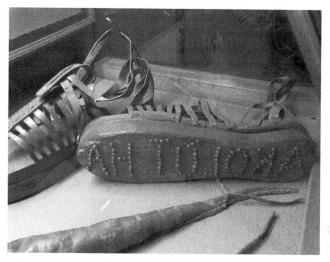

Sandals saying, "Follow Me". Image generously provided by Museum of Sex Machines in Prague.

That's footprint pheromone, surely?

The pheromone the bees use to spread Nasonov and to show which flowers they have already pollinated. "Follow me" is as close an interpretation as you are likely to get for scout bees showing the rest of the swarm the way to the perfect place they've found for their new home.

I mean, it's so uncanny, it's daft, isn't it? It's clearly no coincidence, and since we have archaeological evidence of actual shoes, it proves it's not just a story, either. It's probably the only archaeological evidence that exists that points to something connected to the Melissa playing out in the 3D real world.

The pornai, the street hookers, were taxed in Acrocorinth, and it was their contributions to the wealth of the sanctuary that had ensured it had flourished. A similar belief system was held about Athens. There, authorities report that the sanctuary of Aphrodite Pandemos had been commissioned by Solon, because her image stood in the Agora, but this time the costs of its erection were footed by the hetaerae. In both cases, the glories of the sanctuaries were attributed to Aphrodite's sex workers.

The Sting In The Tale

So, the question I think we must ask ourselves is this...

If Aphrodite is the abortionist, or even the goddess in charge of contraception, how did *she* end up with so many kids? Even if we just count hers and Mars' children that's eight! I think it might have been 16 in total from all her different dalliances.

I mean, it's almost as if she wants to rub her husband Hephaestus's face in it.

It's quite abhorrent really. It's almost as revolting as I felt when I read Herodotus and his aspersions about every woman having to have sex before their wedding.

But I guess you're allowed to behave that way if you're the Queen Bee. Relevantly, the queen can repeatedly sting as many times as she likes, and it won't kill her. It's not unusual for several princesses to hatch together, and it's the job of the first one hatched to sting all the others to death. Very warrior queen. It's survival of the fittest which is nature's way of ensuring the strength of the hive.

Her four to five year life far exceeds that of the 45ish days of a worker bee, who will die if she stings, because her barb lodges into its victim and wrenches her abdomen from her thorax as she pulls away.

The maiden voyage of the virgin princess, though, that's what's wondrous. It is really quite magnificent. It's her sexual appetite, the sovereignty that makes her queen.

Anatomically, she is clearly quite different from a worker. She is longer and bigger. Nevertheless, she can fly and navigate with the same amazing skills as any forager bee can.

Strange, actually, for a creature who will spend so much of her life hidden inside in the dark, but this flying urge to find the sun is exceptionally helpful when she finally goes outside to mate.

Somewhere between five and 14 days after she hatches (a queen hatches at 15-16 days) she leaves the hive and soars towards the sun. It is during this flight of around 600ft, that she will meet drones from many other colonies which, of course, protects the genetic integrity of the hive.

The drones head off for congregation areas which, in my opinion, are absolutely remarkable things.

Each year, male bees head off to the *exact* same place to wait for virgin queens. Usually near a tree growing alone in a field.

Think about how strange that is. Drones die after they have mated, and winter bees kick any unsuccessful ones out to die in the cold, preserving the hive for the females. Thus, there aren't any drones that live for two years to pass on the information of where they should all meet. Nevertheless, every year, the drones *know* where to wait for the princesses.

It's thought they probably navigate by geomagnetic lines, but little more than that is known yet, except that they visit 20 or so sites in a day navigating by landmarks and the sun. Regardless of the process involved, those really are oracle bees, potentially the priests of Apollo.

Only the drones who can fly high enough can mate with her and she typically mates with about 15 in a day. Each one penetrating her, then losing his endophallus, sacrificing himself and falling to his death. The next one comes in, pulls out his predecessor's phallus and then mates with her again.

If necessary, she may take more mating flights to seek out even more males. Each successive mating flight lasts between about five and 30 minutes, depending on how fast she finds drones, and how favourable the weather is toward her.

The warmer the day, the more drones will be flying. In which case, she'll stay out longer if conditions seem favourable.

In some cases, she'll travel huge distances in the hope of finding good drones to mate with in the congregation areas. In theory, sometimes a queen might travel up to six miles to mate, but couples usually pair up around a mile from the hive. The fate of the drone is sealed. Once he has ejaculated, he falls Icarus-like to his death.

Incredibly, from that series of flights the young queen will store up to 70 million sperm from multiple drones in her spermatheca. She will use this advisedly, from now on carefully pondering, "To fertilise, or not to fertilise?" then laying, as previously said, up to 2000 eggs to turn into bees each day.

Isn't she marvellous? The beauty of the animal kingdom, but can you imagine if a woman acted that way?

You just wouldn't, would you? It would be so scandalous. Can you imagine what people would say? We pour scorn on men for deriding women, and as for women saying it…?

Well, that kind of slut-shaming is just not on.

You know, I've always thought of myself as quite an emancipated female. I choose to be monogamous, but if someone else opts for a different lifestyle, that's OK with me. If you had asked me if I would judge another woman for making choices like Aphrodite had, I'd say no, I wouldn't. Well, not that much anyway! It's their business after all. What's it got to do with me?

And I genuinely thought that was true.

But here, let me show you something.

How did you feel about Herodotus and his story about the women in Ishtar's temple? What did you feel about the stories of sexual prostitution?

I can remember the feeling of disgust I felt in my stomach, that this writer seemed to have twisted things to create some kind of anti-Pagan narrative to support the church.

Do you recall the sensation?

Here I'll post it again for you to read:

Every woman born in the country must once in her life go and sit down in the precinct of Venus and there have sex with a stranger. Many of the wealthier sort, who are too proud to mix with the others, drive in covered carriages to the precinct, followed by a goodly train of attendants, and there take their station. But the larger number seat themselves in the holy enclosure with wreaths of string about their heads... and the strangers pass along them to make their choice.

A woman who has taken her seat is not allowed to come home till one of the strangers throws a silver coin into her lap and takes him with her beyond the holy ground. When he throws the coin, he says these words: "The Goddess Mylitta prosper thee." (Venus is called Mylitta by the Assyrians.) The silver coin might be any size; it cannot be refused, for that is forbidden by law, since once it is thrown it is sacred. The woman goes with the first man who throws her money and rejects no-one. When she has gone with him, and so satisfied The Goddess, she returns home, and from that time forth no gift however great will prevail with her. Such of the women who are tall and beautiful are soon released, but others who are ugly have to stay a long time before they can fulfil the law. Some have waited three or four years in the precinct.

Let me ask you, is he talking about Babylonian brides or bees?

Most certainly, he is describing a parallel ritual mimicking the queen flight... he even says how they call her Mylitta – Melissa – bee. She cannot refuse any silver donation, and she must bank it for the rest of her days.

I can't tell you how much this hurts me, because if I am right, then that undoes hundreds of beautiful theses that have fought for women's rights who claim that it can't be. To me, suggesting that those may be wrong feels like a crime against the sisterhood. I stand by it though. That's the nuptial flight of a Melissa.

Oddly, seen through this lens, the practice itself no longer offends me!

I choose to hope they did it through choice, and everything in this research and practice makes me convinced these women were born naturally hypersexual, probably relished being brought to orgasm dozens of times a day, and this service to the community was something they chose to do.

Woman as emancipated and sexual queen, in control of her sovereignty. Of course, the patriarchy had to crush that. Amongst all these intricate comparisons with the hive, it makes absolutely no sense that their sovereign being would be chaste. Further, if the priestess stood in her proxy, neither would she have been chaste either. The priestess was always chosen for her likeness to the goddess, and this one was a hypersexual fertile being, who was different from the others, so had to be born that way with a natural propensity towards sex.

What I will say though, is it makes sense of the Babylonian *hiero gamos*, the sacred marriage, atop of the ziggurat, high above everything in the warmth of the sun. It makes sense of the incestuous royalties, and indeed the arduous climbs to the sanctuaries at Acrocorinth and Eryx too. But to my mind, the idea of a sexual rite taking place in the darkness of the night-time ritual in the telesterion at Eleusis seems much less likely to be. The authorities are clear, the Eleusinian rites belong to Demeter and her priestesses are bees. Bees do not mate in dark, cramped spaces; they soar towards the sun.

If I had to guess what the Heiro Gamos rite of the polis was, I'd suggest it may have been enacted by the *Archon Basileus* and the *Basilinna*. Basilinna means "queen" and it was a ceremonial position held by the wife of the *Archon*. In earlier days, the archon had been a tribal leader, kingly person, but by the time of the Athenians was more of a mayoral figure whose job it was to arrange festivities and presumably his wife functioned as priestess.

The most important duty of the Basilinna is thought to have been to participate in a sacred marriage to Dionysos. The ritual is believed to have taken place as part of the Anthesteria, in late February, early March time, at the Boukoleion, near the Prytaneion which was the seat of Athenian government.

Most scholars consider this rite would have happened on the second day of the festival ("Choes") where an enigmatic drinking-party took place. Contestants competed in silence, draining a nine-pint measure of wine. Slaves were included in the ritual and were entitled to take a share. Children were given miniature choes (the name of the jug they slugged from) as toys, and "first Choes" was a landmark moment.

In some ways though, it makes me wonder if this is even more complex than a marriage as we know it. Its date would align it, in nature, to the first blooms appearing on the ground and the bees going out to drink the first nectar. It's their return with new pollen that signals the queen to start laying, and of course that marks the rebirth of the drones so that they in turn will be able to perpetuate life by crowning new queens.

Ludwig Deubner proposed a full reconstruction of the ceremony, where Dionysos was processed to the sanctuary at Limnai to be wed to the Basilinna; the Basilinna and Dionysos were then accompanied in procession to the Boukoleion, where the marriage was consummated, with the Archon Basileus playing the part of Dionysos.

The party was accompanied by a set of fourteen elderly priestesses who are referred to as the *gererai*. The Basilinna was responsible for administering an oath to these priestesses, who had apparently been appointed by the Archon Basileus.

That the festival takes place right in the first days of spring, and that the gererai were elderly women, seems to speak to those bees who have overwintered the hive. Winter bees live for six months, four times longer than their summer compatriots.

No evidence has ever been found of who these priestesses were or what their function was, but in *The Buzz about Bees*, a fabulous book about bee training flights, J. Tautz has this to say: *"[...] groups of older bees in afternoons preceded virgin queens' mating flights..."*

Chapter 15

Entry into the Hive

After spending about eighteen months writing reams from academic papers, I began to suspect something was lurking beneath the surface that I still didn't have all the data to intuit. There was nothing else written as far as I could tell. It was clear that if I was set on finding out what a priestess really was, I needed to meet and learn from one. I would say my first stroke of luck was given to me by a friend who lives in Glastonbury.

Over dinner, Jan asked how I was getting on with the research and casually dropped the statement, "Of course, you do know the priestesses at Glastonbury call themselves Melissa?"

"No, Jan," I said, taken aback, "I did not know that…"

That there may be Melissae in England was fascinating to me. As it happens, these Bee Women are the guardians of the only Pagan sanctuary in Britain.

Getting one to talk to me was hard though, mainly because I wasn't even sure what I wanted to ask them. It seemed a bit rude to just email and ask for the secrets to their universe, so I held back. There must be some better way.

I've come to realise that the bees really do reorganise the universe if you ask them to, and I think maybe Google might also be run by bees. It's the only way I can explain that after nearly two years of making the search engine groan under pressure of myriad queries about the Melissae… one day a company popped up, right by me, here in Shropshire. Jennifer Naylor is a Magdalene Melissa who runs a business called *Land of Milk and Honey* in Oswestry. Jen is also an aromatherapist as well as being a sound healer specialising in a modality called Naked Voice. She also offers a yearlong training to become a Melissa priestess.

She works with the Divine Feminine outside of the parameters of any set pantheon, but the cycle of sabbats she teaches is informed by Celtic tradition. This felt like it should be helpful to me, a descendant of the Bruce clan, living on the borders of England and Wales, in theory, I guess my blood could be construed as fairly Celtic...

Jen's name does not feature highly in this book, not because she didn't teach me anything; for the opposite reason, actually. She taught me the flow of the hive year and how it ties in with changes that take place within the energies influencing the priestess. Anytime an observation comes up about something falling at a time of the year, that credit should go to Jen.

One warm afternoon, quarantined at home in lockdown protection to prevent the spread of the COVID-19 pandemic, I was sitting in my beautiful arbour, surrounded by cushions with a bumblebee crawling up my arm. I'd rescued no fewer than four from the paddling pool, that day, after they'd tried to take a drink and then not been able to get out again. This bee was huge, and almost entirely black. Every now and then she'd buzz a bit as she fanned in an attempt to dry herself off. She seemed quite besotted by me, this bee. No matter how many times I tried to encourage her to be with her friends on the lavender or lavatera, she made it very clear she would much prefer to enjoy the taste of the sweat glistening on my arm.

So, I sat quietly, headphones on, so as not to disturb her and trawled through YouTube looking for clues. I came across a podcast interview with a lady called Ariella Daly from a company called Honey Bee Wild. As Ariella talked about "all-things-bee", she began to speak about how she had come from America to England to study bee shamanism at the Sacred Trust, under a woman by the name of Naomi Lewis who had, in turn, spent time learning from women influenced by Lithuanian Melissae. She teaches the course to handpicked students where Simon Buxton also teaches shamanism.

Ariella is a very softly spoken, gentle creature with a mellifluous voice full of mystery. That she had trained at the Sacred Trust seemed almost too good to be true. I visited her website to find out more, only to discover she also taught disciplines influenced by the Path of Pollen.

To answer the very obvious question before we go on: why seek out an American to teach you, when the main centre is in England? Most of the Sacred Trust courses had waiting lists, and face-to-face workshops were out of the question because we were locked down anyway. Truth be told though, the final part of Simon's initiation, him spending days buried alive, scared the pants off me! Both process and person terrified me. I didn't relish being asked to do that, and any route that meant I didn't have to be covered in soil seemed better to me!

Ariella's core teaching is dream weaving, as was performed in the sanctuaries of Asklēpiós, the god of medicine. That was a challenge in itself, because after having terrifying nightmares as a child, I had learnt not to dream. Needless to say, I was a tad worried I might be wasting my time. I emailed Ariella, asked if it would be worth joining the course and was open about the book being my reason for doing it. In her usual way she was concise, sweet, and clear; she was up for it if I was. It was worth a try.

Now, I am sure any of my overseas colleagues probably saw the next part coming a mile off, but I didn't. As far as I was concerned, the classes fit perfectly into my schedule, starting around the time I usually break from writing to do the housework at one o'clock. The morning of the first class arrived and I checked my times only to realise... no, Liz... that's one o'clock in the morning!

So, through the autumn and winter of 2020, I'd powernap on Monday afternoons and then head up early to get my head down in the spare bedroom. At just after midnight, I switched on the electric blanket, crept downstairs to arm myself with warm drinks and hot water bottles. On entry into my office which is a dark and draughty shed, I climbed into sleeping bags and blankets then wrapped myself in a big old black crocheted shawl. One can't be too careful you know, there are no prizes for being cold!

Ariella's courses are done over Zoom. Since no-one turns on their cameras, disembodied voices floated in the dark. Thirteen of us: the bee mistress, plus two sets of six apprentices, worked together to weave and interpret dreams. Together we learned how to visualise the womb becoming the head of a bee, our fallopian tubes as its antennae, its proboscis reaching down through the Earth, to where the bees take the souls of the dead. I have never been so tired in my life or loved anything quite so much.

It was fascinating to hear how accomplished people were at dreaming, how much symbology was encoded within them and how much knowledge could be gleaned from them. It took courage, I will confess, to allow myself to begin dreaming again, after a lifetime of hiding from it, but as I allowed my brain to register the pictures, I became enchanted.

So, when that initial course ended, and the opportunity to work on a one-to-one basis with Ariella arose, I jumped at it. Likewise, I then got in contact with the former members of the dream group to try to set up our own hive. As it stands, there are now only five of us in the dreaming hive, but I stand by the maxim that it's our quality not quantity that counts!

Large chunks of Melissae training are taught via *Knowledge Lectures*, which are quite the most beautiful thing. I think it's probably what made me fall in love with the tradition. Both Ariella, and Jen who is the High Priestess of my Magdalene Melissa hive, are incredibly clever at speaking with languid bee metaphor. Their words ooze the sweetness of honey. It took me a while to get the hang of receiving Knowledge Lectures, because it required me to put down my pen. Anyone who has sat near me at a conference will know how much I like to take notes! One of the first things I had to learn, was to listen in a hugely different way. Instead of operating from the second brain in my head, I needed to hear things with the first brain, the womb space.

For the longest time, I couldn't actually move my attention down to my womb. I would feel it come to a gridlock standstill at my solar plexus. In the dreams that accompanied these difficulties, witches burned, their legs perpetually melting into the flames. I began to believe this fear of being seen could be connected with the acid reflux that scorched my throat. Written down, that seems banal, yet this awful fear of revealing secrets would become a horrifying bitterness that affected my power to eat. Oddly, in the middle of a weave one night, unaided by any mention of my digestive condition, I was given details of pungent herbs for acid reflux as part of my dream mirror.

Eventually, I gained the courage to get my attention down, but not without developing an addiction to aniseed balls. I literally ate the whole of Ludlow's supply and then they couldn't get them in because of lockdown so I had to buy kilo bags just to get by!

At the core of the dream-work teaching is the idea that the bees inhabit an invisible golden dream net that wraps the world and the cosmos (look at Delphi's omphalos), and that when the priestesses dream together, with intention, a divine messaging system begins to form. Over time, it becomes clear that this is true; that the dream weave is indeed an arc of combined and related information that comes together to create pictures which can be woven into oracles.

The dream weave reflects the collective unconsciousness of the many.

One of the key meditations of the tradition is **The Walk of Infinite Flight**. The apprentice is taught the rudiments of it in a Knowledge Lecture and then sent away to just do it over and over, always noting down their feelings, thoughts, and epiphanies.

Teacher of Bee Shamanism, Simon Buxton, described it in an interview he did with Karen Sawyer for her book, *Soul Companions*.

I invite you to try it... put 10 minutes aside, and, as a Total Act, walk the figure 8. What will typically be discovered is that after just 10 minutes you will find that your level of mental clarity and your sense of balance and well-being have been heightened to a noticeable degree. Simply by walking that figure – the figure that was a gift to us from the bees – has the effect of bringing a beautiful harmony and balance between the left hand and the right hand sides of the brain. The Path of Pollen walks equally in an impeccably balanced fashion, both the left hand and right hand paths, accessing the intellect and intuition evenly, and seeking to balance the feminine and the masculine within the physical body and within the psyche of the individual. One of the gifts that the hive has brought us is the opportunity to create a balanced life constantly exploring infinity itself.

I must tell you this story:

One afternoon in July, The Silent One arrived from work later than usual. As he came in the door he said, "I don't know what's going on with your hive, but there's hundreds of them outside. You might want to take a look. I think something might have upset them."

I quickly donned my shoes, racing down the steps in a panic, fearful they were swarming without me saying goodbye. He was right, something strange *was* definitely going on. There were dozens at the entrance and dozens more swirling round, higher and higher in the air, seemingly emulating the shape of the pond. I suspected there might be something in the water they didn't like, but there didn't seem to be anything amiss.

I have a chair by the hive, to watch or sit and meditate with them. I asked them if they were OK, and for a moment, I speculated they might be responding to being robbed (bees do rob honey from other hives), but it was clear to me they were calm. They didn't seem angry at all. Half a dozen bees sat like pigeons on the hive roof fanning, bums in the air, wafting as much Nasonov as they could muster. The flying bees swirled round in arcs, flew back to the entrance and went straight back in. Then another came out and did the same. Naturally, it was impossible to know if they were the same bees. It was beautiful and enigmatic to watch, they seemed calm, and I didn't *think* they were swarming since these bees seemed to be calling them *in*.

I like to imagine that my bees like me to drum to them or tang with my singing bowl, so I went and got them from the shed, just in case that would calm them somehow. When I returned, a majestic-looking fly with incredible rust-coloured markings and huge staring eyes had also appeared on the end of the roof. The guard bees soon saw him off, but I questioned if perhaps he might have been the robber who had found his way in to feast upon their honey.

Nevertheless, I hummed with them, tanging various bowls until the chaos had calmed down and most of them had found their way back in.

Sheepishly, looking at my watch, I realised guiltily that The Silent One's dinner would be quite tardy, this night!

Later, when everyone else had headed off to bed for the night, I started to think about their strange behaviour again, searching the web for explanations of what I might have seen. I didn't fancy my chances of finding anything to my search of "Bees buzzing madly outside the hive", but to my surprise I found a plausible answer straight away. We had witnessed the forager's training flight.

On regular evenings around dinner time, about two hours before sundown, the trainees practise orienting themselves to the sun. They fly out of the hive, turn 180 degrees, head back, then do it again, creating these ever-increasing arcs in the sky. The bees on the roof were secreting Nasonov to imprint on them and teach them the way back to the hive.

I was so delighted to have witnessed it and to have been able to sit for so long and watch. Closing the laptop and heading off to bed, I couldn't wait to tell The Silent One in the morning what we'd seen.

Next morning, Parsnip was back. She'd been absent for a while. Giggling as she does… "Did you see it?"

"I did! I loved it!"

"So, what is it?"

"The Orientation Flight," I told her, smug at my quick recollection.

"And…?"

"And, what?" I frowned, disappointed at how unimpressed she seemed.

"It's the Orientation Flight and…? Well, you know what you need to do today then."

I'd got an incredibly busy day ahead, presenting an online lecture and then cleaning for an estate agent to come and value our house, in the hope that, after ten years here, we might be able to buy it. I groaned audibly at the prospect of trying to find a training flight in the myths. I scanned the places I suspected it might be, but nothing jumped out.

That morning, the hive was business as normal when I checked on the girls, so I headed back to the cottage to start to clear up. I'd left the webpage I'd been reading the night before open, and seeing it with fresh eyes, Parsnip's assignment was now easy.

Young bees walk out of the hive, fly a short distance in front, turn by 180 degrees so that they are facing the hive, then hover back and forth in arcs. After a few moments, the orientation flight becomes

characterised by the ever increasing circles around and above the
hive and after a few minutes the bee returns to its hive without
carrying any pollen or nectar.[65]

That's an almost exact description of the Walk of Infinite Flight.

And here, as the bees do their own training flight, older bees rest on the roof secreting Nasonov, the bee pheromone that smells the same as Melissa. Bizarrely, six of them, each time I've seen it, which is the same number of apprentices you have working with the Bee Mistress.

The orientation flights tend to take place on warm windless
afternoons. Interestingly, on these flights, "foragers to be" take
the opportunity to void their faeces, as they had not had a chance
to cleanse previously.[66]

I love the last sentence of the trial because the practice is so dynamic, that it does indeed clear so much crap! Some days, I can go from feeling like I am on my knees with stress, to soaring above the clouds. It's such a beautiful practice. I have been doing it daily for about a year now and had had absolutely no clue what it was. Whether that is its ritual, who can say, but I like to imagine that it is, that I too am learning the skills of how to orient myself with the life source of the universe and that the Melissae elders sit in sentry to lead me home. It comforts me and makes me overflow with love.

Sia's "Courage To Change" became my mantra and introduction to every Walk I did, to remind myself there were other women doing this practice openly, who were alive.

Over time I have come to think of doing The Walk more as a method of "patrolling" and see it as a vital part of developing oracular knowing. Research shows that eusocial insects, including honey bees, patrol comb as a method of gathering global information. They spend vast amounts of time walking to and fro feeling vibrations communicated through their feet and sensing pheromones. Interestingly, from my own point of view middle-aged bees walk the furthest entering every work area gathering information about all aspects of both the hive, but also the outside (as yet unseen) world at large.[67]

Very little information is given directly to the apprentice. What is imparted is dripped in small amounts. Knowledge Lectures are delivered to the trainee bee with her eyes closed. It's not written down, and if it is, it must be regurgitated before being recapitulated. In other words, chew it over, allow your own alchemical vessel to change it before you pass it on. The requirements to recall so many details definitely improve certain aspects of your memory, but there is something uncannily wonderful about the way they are told. Words drip like honey into hidden places in the body, igniting thoughts that drift on the waves of wonder. In the darkness, your mind fights to keep up with the strange strings of words and creates all manner of pictures and constructions. How one apprentice conceives of something will be different to how the next one does. It's that individuality that creates the magic.

So many of the aspects of the Melissa are disparate, but what stands at the very centre of the teaching is the sacred capacities of the womb space, and the Melissa's journey to control her own necktary (with a k), her inner garden of flowers which she trains to flower, spin, and drip. Different to the Eastern chakra system, the Path of Pollen uses the Western tradition of eight energy centres, each with many colour, sound, planetary and endocrine correlations.

The priestesses work on a system of roses and stars using several totems, including spider, snake and, of course, the bee. The Bee Mistress is deemed to be mistress of her own laboratory, able to secrete and control her internal body fluids at will. Then by way of ingesting the might of sun, fire, and vital Earth energies the Melissa uses breathwork and arcane meditations to revivify both herself and the world around her. At all times on her journey towards mastery, she seeks spiritual knowledge or gnosis.

Frustratingly, the apprentice is never told where she is expected to end up. There is no sense of "This is what we are learning to do", which was exasperating when I was trying to understand who the priestess was. It took a long time to realise the seeking *was* the point, but as the journey towards "enlightenment", to steal a Buddhist term, unravels, the priestess learns many things about herself, and about the seen and unseen worlds as she comes into a new way of being. Concurrently, her meditation practices begin to move etheric energies and fluids around her system.

From an Apollonian point of view, it is perhaps easiest to think of these fluids as secretions of the endocrine system. That would be correct, but for every gland there is also an unseen Dionysian component, a dripping, a vapour that, with much practice, can be moved and used at will. This etheric blood is recognisable in Greek mythology as ichor, the blood that runs through the veins of the gods.

Many of the characters we encounter in the myths are called nymphs. We can view this term in several ways: a nymph is the second stage of a bee, the larva who has yet to develop wings. In the context of the ancient world at large, a nymph may be a woman who has yet to wed. In the Path of Pollen, however, we should view these women as advanced priestesses who had become mistresses of their nectaries, and as such, had learnt how to control them to unleash ichor around their bodies. In this context, we can see how nymphs might have received their apotheosis into Goddess, that they have learnt to circulate this Elixir of Life. Lastly, nymphs also have a more mythic definition of women who were human, but seemingly had the power to commune with and to shapeshift into animals, plants, and trees. Every interpretation applies, and it behoves the apprentice to contemplate that there may be instances where things can simultaneously exist in more than just one state at once.

Whilst clearly within the tradition there would have been myriad different healers, astronomers, midwifes, dancers… it is this work on the necktary – reminiscent of how the worker bee which is ordinarily sterile can control her own sexuality – that most resembles the hive.

In the tradition, it is thought there are two types of Melissa, one who dutifully collects pollen and nectar (note the different spelling betrays the interpretation as *probably* being about the insect) and takes them back to the hive. The other type is a far more sensual being who comes into ecstatic union with the flower, drowning in the bliss of the fragrance. Oddly, for an aromatherapist who languishes in the beauty of the aroma of the plant, I was surprised to find that I do not belong to the latter group, although through the following pages we will meet some who most certainly are.

We can further divide those Melissae again. This time into three groups, The Spinners, The Wise Maidens, and the Fae. Only when a Melissa has achieved full mastery of her necktary, will she earn the title of Fae. Fae are shapeshifters and powerful magicians.

Perhaps the most famous example of these was Morgan la Fae, or Morgana. Today, Morgan's spirit can be felt in Glastonbury, the modern-day Avalon, still calling to sacred women. Interestingly she tends the waters, bringing her priestesses to the lake. When she was first described in the 12th century text, *Vita Merlini* (1150 CE), we were told she held the knowledge of herbs and healing ointments, that she had second sight, and possessed the ability to shapeshift. The stories tell how she could manifest "new wings like Daedalus" who also was not born with wings but fashioned them out of wax.[68] Interpretations of what this might mean differ. Was she someone who knew how to relinquish humanness to obtain the power of flight? Or was she faery queen? In my opinion, it seems ever more possible to suspect both.

Morgan is described as having wings (that may have been artificial, but it's difficult to discern) and seemingly had the ability to remove them at will. Interestingly, we can see how she may be related to the water nymphs or may actually be a water bee. As an aside, it is also recorded that she taught her sisters mathematics, which also seems to appear as a theme when we read about Melissa Delphis, the Pythia.[64]

Chapter 16

Private Moments

The first week of April 2021 saw stunning weather in Shropshire. The sun was warm, and flowers were bursting through everywhere. One morning, as I walked, listening to the churn of the river and enjoying the flowers shooting in the gardens, something caught my eye, on the bank at the side of the pavement.

Amongst the celandines, a black bug scurried, then another popped out of her hole, and yet another. I watched, fascinated, as these pretty insects with grey hairy collars and slender, elegant wings teemed out of their nest. Within seconds, dozens of them were rushing around between the weeds' dark green leaves.

I resolved to look them up when I got home, but busy-ness prevented me from doing so. Then in the evening, my mother-in-law rang from the Vienne, in France, to give us the sad news that her husband had died about half an hour after she'd left the hospital that evening. After several months of being ill, he had finally found peace from his struggle.

We began the complex job of getting Darrell and his brother over to the continent during restrictions and France's curfew. There being no flights, the lads decided to go on the Eurotunnel and drive. While navigating all the pages of requirements we had to fill, a newsflash popped up with more sad news. The Duke of Edinburgh was dead.

It would be a few days later, when finally, he was off on his way, that I would find time to look up what the insects were that I'd seen hatching from their nests. *Melecta albifrons* better known as Common Mourning Bees.

The bees truly were harbingers of death.

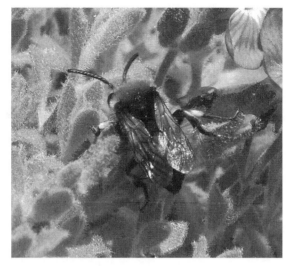

Common Mourning Bee. Photograph by Gail Hampshire.

Chapter 17

Orthi Petra and the Minoan Priestesses

The Minoan civilization predates the rites of Eleusis by around 1500 years and shows clear connections to veneration of bees.

Much of the knowledge we have about the Minoans comes from an archaeologist by the name of Sir Arthur Evans, an eminent Oxford scholar and guardian of my most beloved museum, the Ashmolean. The "Ash" is chock full of the most incredible ancient Greek artefacts, thanks, in all probability, to Evans and his exploits.

The story tells of how he had purchased a stone engraved with a labryrs – a double axe – that had encouraged him to purchase the piece of land where it had been found.

A colleague of Evans, Minos Kalokairinos, had originally uncovered the first hints of the Palace of Knossos on Crete in 1878. Finally, in 1900, Evans began to excavate the site that he and his team would continue to study for the next 35 years. Knossos, home to the Snake Goddess entombed for millennia; a place, he concluded must have been the Labyrinth – because the word means "Home of the Double Axe". Since the labyrinth was home of the Minotaur, he christened the name of the people he was studying as "Minoan".

Cult agents of Knossos celebrated around a strange altar, shaped like a pair of bull's horns that Evans referred to as the "Horns of Consecration".

He explained his fascination with the original labrys he'd found came from his knowledge that priests serving at Delphi were sometimes known by the title *Labryades* – Servants of The Double Axe. Thus, he concluded that there may have been some kind of connection between what happened in this Minoan cultic setting and what may have taken place, hundreds of years later at Delphi.

Interestingly though, even though the priests held the Labryades name, it is always the *priestesses* who are depicted as wielding the axe. Evans felt sure that it had something to do with a tree cult, or maybe that some kind of pillar was worshipped.

Perhaps it's only to be expected that history might provide frustratingly few answers to Evans' questions. Priestesses devoutly kept silent vows and took secrets they knew to their graves. Those graves have often been robbed when found, visual clues dismantled, and all manner of context taken away.

It's almost impossible to find an intact tomb.

Almost.

But let me tell you, as a Melissa, I'm starting to realise that anything to do with the bee cultus is possible....

Records show that Evans had done some superficial surveys of the area around Eleutherna, decided there was nothing of significance there and moved on. Unbeknownst to him, beneath his feet was perhaps one of the most remarkable snapshots of human history to ever be discovered, a necropolis that had been in consistent use for almost 3000 years.

Dorian warriors from ancient Macedonia had conquered and colonised Eleutherna sometime between 1100 and 900 BCE. They controlled vast territories and it's not difficult to see why they would have wanted to put roots down in the area, surrounded as it still is, by unparalleled beauty. They built their sanctuary on a high slope, almost smack bang on the island's geographical centre. To the east were iron mines, and to the north, lush grazing lands and, what would eventually become, the bustling city port of Cydonia. To the south, a heavily forested area which proffered precious timber for boatmaking and construction. This is the area where Knossos, and neighbouring Heraklion would come to be built. The land was rich with herbs. Flowers and medicinal plants were frequented by bees who made bountiful amounts of beeswax which could be used to make candles and subsequently also became invaluable for casting metal. We mustn't forget, of course, all that exquisite honey.

From high on the hillside, a spectacular vista of greenery leads the eye out to sea, and in antiquity, Eleutherna would have been flanked by Crete's two most important ports, Panormos and Stavromenos.

Crete is Greece's fifth largest island and covers an area of around 160 miles. At its narrowest, the distance across the island is just over seven miles. At its widest, about 37. In ancient times, the island formed the crossroads between the East and West, attracting merchants laden with goods and ideas from Asia, Africa, and Europe.

About ten miles from Eleutherna, is Mount Ida, Crete's highest mountain which rises just over 8000ft above sea level. The mountain was deemed to be sacred to Rhea. The Idaean cave, where she was believed to have birthed Zeus, sits upon one of its flanks. It was here that the god was said to have been fed by the goat nymph Amalthea, or perhaps the Melissae. As the child fussed, the mythical warrior Kouretes guarded the cave, loudly clashing their copper shields like cymbals to hide the sound of his cries lest his father Cronus discover he'd been duped. I like to imagine an accompaniment of cicadas noisily clattering their own tiny tympanums besides them.

One of the Kouretes, Elefthere would eventually give his name to Eleutherna. Interestingly, the mother of the Kouretes was considered to be Cybele and she, too, had a hill called Mount Ida made sacred to her. This one is found in Turkey, in ancient Anatolia.

The land surrounding Eleutherna is indescribably lovely, lush, green, and majestic. The site is encircled by olives, carob, cypresses, and oaks which burst from creamy coloured rock set against azure skies. Most assuredly, one can see why the goddess might have felt drawn to it.

The Idaean Cave has competition for Zeus' birth legend though, as some sources relate how he may have been born in the Dictean Cave. This one is perhaps more reminiscent of another cave set aside for Eileithyia, the great goddess of childbirth, whose own child was born into a cave which housed a stalactite in the middle.

Honestly, though, it's not difficult to imagine a deity being born anywhere on the exquisite isle of Crete. Not only is it stunning, in a time where caves were considered the vagina of the Great Mother, it's not surprising it became such a hallowed place. Apart from those of religious and historical significance, another 4500 caves have been mapped. Famously, light glistens from myriad sparkling crystals in the Sfendoni Cave, chock full of stalagmites and stalactites.

Also of interest might be the Labyrinth Cave, which some scholars believe may have inspired the story of the Minotaur. The labyrinthine structure is artificially made, full of corridors that can run as long as 2.5km long, leading into rooms and chambers that go nowhere. Actually, it's a quarry that provided stone for palaces built in the area. The limestone is prime building material, as well as being wonderful to sculpt with, and would have been in plentiful demand. Some scholars suspect the Theseus story may have been an allegory for the mental health of miners sent down there to work.

The island has the most extraordinary geology because it is a subduction zone. In these areas, the edges of tectonic plates shift and move under each other. These plates of the earth's crust move sideways and down, pushing into the mantle of the earth, disturbing the geology of the ground.

An astonishing visual representation of this can be seen at Agia Pavlos where the rocks are striated in a kind of chevron pattern, where competent and incompetent materials have been alternately compressed. I am reminded of the honeycomb structures made by wild bees, and whimsically, I imagine how easy it must have been to imagine souls pushing their way back out of the ground. I wondered if they looked and saw the rocks as proof that perhaps, in the past, people had.

Geologists believe these compressional forces began around 40 million years ago and are responsible for the vast mountains and valleys and the island's frequent earthquakes. Crete experiences at least one minor quake a year, and history testifies to several larger ones having happened during the past millennium, some of which have been accompanied by tsunamis.

In Bettany Hughes' TV series, *Greek Odyssey*, she visits a live archaeological dig on Crete, only to come face to face with the grim discovery of the body of a young maiden who seems to have been sacrificed in a bid to appease the gods in the midst of one awful earthquake.

The most catastrophic event is thought to have happened in the 15th century BCE when the volcano on Santorini exploded, possibly leading to the demise of the Minoan civilization.

The name *Orthi Petra* means "Standing Stone" and relates to the tall pillar found at the centre of the necropolis. Reminiscent of an Egyptian obelisk, it verifies Aristotle's narrative that the Cretans and Spartans were unusual in that they chose to venerate their dead within the confines of the city. The bridge that marks its entrance is unsettlingly reminiscent of a hexagon.

In the words of the Director of Excavations, Nicholas Stampolidis, *"the site stands out like a huge, petrified ship,"* the two galleys of the vessel having been gouged out by running streams surrounding it, which gush in the rainy season.

That the architecture of the necropolis was formed in the shape of a ship is fascinating. Ship symbology in the bee story is far reaching and complex.

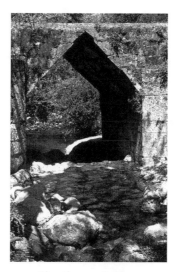

Eleutherna Bridge.

In Egyptology, many solar barges have been recovered from tombs, including Khufu's boat that was discovered under the Great Pyramid. Indeed, no fewer than seven boat pits have been found in close proximity to it. The Solar Barge transported the *ba* of the resurrected Pharoah across the skies on his voyage to collect the souls of the dead. The ba, of course, was worshipped as Osiris Apis.

In a book of essays dedicated to the memory of the Welsh poet Iorwerth C. Peate, English writer Osbert Sitwell recounts an amusing story from his East Anglian childhood.

His family had a butler, he says, who used to point at clouds, solemnly sighing: "the big Norwegian Bishops." Presumably, the family thought it a tad peculiar, but delightful enough that they were able to recall it years later when they'd heard a similar saying. Somehow the butler had misheard it. Sitwell describes how they'd discovered this saying should have not been Bishops, but *Bee skeps* or *Bee ships*.

The saying, from Norse mythology, was that souls of the dead are represented as bees and were supposed to traverse the sky in what was specifically termed as a bee-ship.

He writes:

And it should be pointed out that the old straw-plaited skep could easily be considered as an analogue of a well-rounded cumulus cloud. Moreover, Virgil compares a swarm of bees to a dark cloud being drawn across the sky by the wind.[68]

In the Trojan stories, it was said that ships were despatched from Hyria. But Hesychius revealed that *Hyron* (the singular form of the Cretan word Hyria) had two meanings, either a swarm of bees or a beehive.[44] It's almost as if bees were sent from Hyria, and as we know, the Greeks too believed bees to be psychopomps of the soul.

Tools, idols, and stone axes have been recovered from the necropolis of Eleutherna, which shows human use from around 3200 BCE. Incredibly the site was in continuous use from the geometric period, through the Archaic, Classical, Hellenistic, and Byzantine periods right up to around 1400 CE. It is a rich source of information, particularly about the Minoan and late bronze age.

The site gives unprecedented insights into how the people of the age buried their dead. When tomb A1K1 was discovered, it revealed the exciting information that the burial site closely echoed the detailed narrative that Homer gave of a funerary ritual in *The Iliad*. Achilles cremated his friend Patroclus on a funeral pyre, and slaughtered prisoners of war to give as grave offerings in retribution for the deaths of his comrades. The burial site revealed, as well as many cremated offerings interred in urns, the unburned skeleton of a man aged around 35 years. His head had been severed from his body, to separate it from his soul. The head had been burned, but his body remained untouched by funeral rites, cast out as if to wander between this world and the other. Like a blossom, fading before its time, he had been deadheaded.

The narrative in *The Iliad* is gruesomely detailed and is shown exactly this way in the burial. Thus, when the story was later recited as one of the key features of the Great Panathenaea in Athens festivities, we now know the Grecians were receiving explicit instructions about how to bury their dead. As Homer had said in the Odyssey:

> *I put you under oath now. Remember me. Don't leave me behind unburied and ungrieved. Cremate me with my panoply and build a tomb for me. For those that haven't been yet to remember...*[69]

There were no acceptable excuses. Regardless of situation, priest or no priest, everyone had to know how to dispose of the dead.

For the most part, men's bodies seem to have been cremated. Elderly women and children were buried inside of huge jars known as *pythoi*. These had originally been thought to have been used by lower born women who perhaps had not had the means for an expensive burial, but this theory was overturned in 2009 when the team uncovered a set of interlocking ceramic vessels, each of varying heights between 5.2ft and 6.5ft, containing richly-adorned women. They seemed to be the remains of a least three generations of one family.

The pythoi were covered with pseudo phalluses that stretched across the tomb like ribs. Buried with them were ceramic vases, bowls, sumptuous gold jewellery including spindles and a beautiful golden bee. In a lecture given by Stampolidis to The Met, an image was shown of the site. Each of the pythoi were pushed into the last, forming a tube, in just the same way that solitary bees make their nests. Each woman had been furnished with everything she would need for what was to come.

Their dresses were embossed with gold that had been laid over their clothes in stripes. The vast riches of gold and semi-precious stones suggest highborn women, probably priestesses.

Then, archaeologists were to discover yet more astonishing evidence of priestesses when a small mausoleum building was unearthed. At its western side, there was an elaborately carved doorway, which was closed with well-fitting slabs. Inside the tomb were four women, thought to be aged 13, 16, 28 and 72; again, all from one family.

The elderly woman appears to have been buried in a sitting position, with the others laid out in descending order, the eldest to the west, then the youngest at the east.

Each of the women had been adorned with scarabs, earrings, bracelets, and bead necklaces, made of the most opulent materials you can imagine, gold, silver, Egyptian blue, amber, quartz, and semi-precious stones.

The collection of golden jewellery is glorious. One piece depicts a goddess, another a Master of The Beasts flanked by two lions. Another has a lion stalking, seemingly ready to pounce. On another, we meet two warriors staring at each other, face to face. They also had a small bronze statuette of a bull, a tiny bronze ladle, and a small saw. Near the middle of the tomb was a table.

In the eastern and slightly northern and southern areas, they unearthed large amphorae that had probably contained some kind of liquid, perhaps wine or olive oil. One amphora was covered by the kind of glass phiale that we see priestesses using to pour libations. Between the table and the amphorae were a variety of exquisite bronze vessels of different sorts, a series of phiale, cups, and a lamp all made from bronze. These were laid in an east-westerly line, and it made me think of how modern Pagan altars would deem that to be the air-water axis. I wondered what they were concocting to boil. There was a disk from a scale still suspended on its chain.

The elderly woman seems to have been mummified in some way and indeed even though she had fallen forward in her chair, when she was found 2700 years later, her nose had remained intact.[70] Although the details of their deaths are unclear to me, the paper about their subsequent forensic research into their bones and teeth seems to suggest a group ritual suicide. The paper is exquisitely poetic, in many places especially this:

Among a few competitive explanatory hypotheses under investigation, a conditional proposition is also explored under the supposition that at a juncture in time embedded in the parchments of Cleo, possibly triggered by a momentous event, and in the ultimate expression of selfless sacrifice, in respectful and obedient conduct bound by moral obligation and the permanent dictates of virtue and conscience, in dedication and loyalty to the lawful and dutiful fulfilment of actions required of particular socio-cultural positions held, and/or in piety, devotion and fealty in a conferred allegiance to the occult existence of the divine, a substance of deleterious influence possibly with a somniferous precursor that had invoked Atropos to act, allowed them in unique fellowship to transcend and to carry on eternally their duties and functions in the asphodel meadows of Hades.

Admittedly we may never know their names, their individual thoughts, their individual responsibilities, their expectations, their hopes and dreams... Yet gleaning on aspects of the esoteric complexities and the emerging apparition of their meaningful relations, at the initial unfolding of this ancient riddle discovered and the narrative deciphered so far, confide not only a nexus to ancestral times and most significant events but also bestow the responsibility to search deeper beyond the extent of the perceived fundamentals, enthused with great anticipation that further interdisciplinary inquiry and long term research based on methodical procedures and careful analysis would shed additional light to the matters at hand on the spirited sequence of events and splendid accomplishments attained by our ancients at Eleutherna.[71]

You would have thought discovering the grave of the priestesses would have pleased me, and in some ways it did, but more it stopped me in my tracks. It made the cult very real and suddenly I no longer needed anyone to remind me these meditations were merely whimsical thoughts.

To these women, 2700 years ago, this was their lives. It was the tenet they lived by.

When I next visited the hive, I asked the bees to thank the Minoan priestesses for their amazing sacrifice, but to tell them, I still really didn't understand it. I'd never be able to summon that kind of courage. Somehow, it seemed to me they had been martyred, or were dying to achieve something, but I really didn't understand what. Endless theories ran through my mind, but I wanted to hear it from them.

One thing you come to realise in Melissa medicine, is never to expect a straight answer. In fact, sometimes I wonder if the labyrinth isn't actually an allegory for priestess training! A question always generates at least three more – and if it is only three, then I count myself lucky! Thus, no-one was more shocked than I when there was just one clear question.

What do the bees do with the queen when she dies?

A simple question.

Not an easy one to get an answer to.

Any search engine enquiry only gave up information about supersedure; how the workers start to feed up new princesses, but there seemed to be a gap... if this was a cult that copied the hive, and there seemed to be fascination with burial... where was the queen's body?

I emailed three of my beekeeping mentors to ask what they had observed.

Three answers the same, but one with a little more detail than the others.

Enough to make me weep.

As we know, undertaker bees take care of the bodies, clearing them out from the hive. The queen receives no special attention, and that can be seen by the fact that sometimes there is nothing left in the debris outside of the hive but a tiny speck of paint that shows where she had been marked.

But how she dies is tragic.

As she ages and weakens, no longer secreting QMP, the workers begin to withhold food. The sustenance they need for the princesses is taken from her. Why feed her now that her worth has gone? Instead, her attendants surround her tightly, smothering her in a group huddle.

I contemplated that may have been what had happened to the elderly priestess. Had her magic begun to fail her, so she had now outgrown her use? The archeo-dental records showed how the youngsters seemed to have had times when food sources had been really low. Had the rains not come? Had she known her power was failing, and suspected a younger woman might do a better job than she?

Was it time to hand over sovereignty at last? Was it possible that her faith was so strong she believed her sacrifice to be enough to appease the sun god? Did she trust in the reward that awaited her in the life ever after?

If so, I envied her depth of certainty. I have never believed in anything that much.

Except, perhaps, in the power of bees.

The story might be even more tragic than that.

I had thought that the term "colony collapse" meant that the hive just died, but that's not necessarily so. What actually happens is the worker bees stage a full-scale walk out. They desert the queen, leaving her with a few attendants, expecting them to fend for themselves. But the attendants are not yet mature enough to gather forage, so those left behind will eventually starve.

The similarity with the tomb chilled me.

Did the community just head off to find new pastures, leaving their beloved priestess behind, no longer believing she had what it took to protect them now, but trusting her enough to accept her suggestion of offering herself up as propitiation for the gods?

Had the harvest been ruined by the scorching sun? Or worse, had plagues of locusts greedily robbed it all? I was surprised to know that locusts aren't a genus in their own right. In fact, it is the heat of the sun that transforms them from harmless grasshoppers into ravenously destructive fiends. As I studied them, I stared at the genus name Orthopter, haunted by the eerie similarity to the necropolis where the priestesses rested at Ortho Petra.

As is the way, sooner or later someone else may have moved in to the area to take the tribe's place, but potentially, for these priestesses at least, their advent would have come too late to save them. I pray that Knossos's poppy goddess smothered them into merciful oblivion.

Chapter 18

The Snake Goddess

Sir Arthur Evans surmised that the palace at Knossos was ruled by a priest-prince surrounded by priestesses. These beautiful priestesses appear on many friezes, especially in the Palace of Knossos, sometimes wielding the double axe, and often wearing a bow tied at the back of their neck, reminiscent of tiny wings.

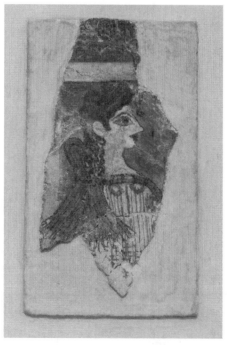

The Minoan priestess fresco known as La Parisienne, wearing the sacral knot bow. Photograph by Jebulon.

His theory of a Prince Priest was based on many suppositions, but pertinently that the "throne room" was painted with griffins which are deemed to be a symbol of The Goddess.

As years have passed, doubt has been cast on some of the conclusions he made. He "renovated" the palace as he believed it would have been. Using his knowledge of Classical Greece as a template, he painted the columns in bright colours for example, as it is believed they would have been in Greece. Nevertheless, there is no proof this was the fashion on Crete a thousand years before that time. So whether their vivid appearance was accurate is uncertain, and further, more recently scholars have proposed they themselves may have been so rustic they were actually upturned trees, the roots holding up the roof.

In reconstructing the frescoes, he used one wall as a template for the others and used that as a guide for repainting what he thought should be underneath, filling the room with griffins. However, that may not have been the artist's original intention and as such we can't be sure certain symbolism wasn't lost in the process.

It is now also clear that an image of the Lily Prince, which the entire supposition of Evans' hypothesis was based upon, is actually made from pieces from three separate frescoes. Later restorations inform the knowledge that men in the pictures had been painted in a red ochre hue, but women were given paler, whiter skin. This now illuminated the discovery that two of the frescoes used to assemble the image of the priest were actually pictures of women and the rope he holds in his hand, which perhaps may suggest some ritual use, may also be part of his invention.

Perhaps, the most famous treasures unearthed at Knossos are the two snake goddess statuettes, now housed in the Heraklion Museum. Thought to be somehow associated with the bee cultus, they date to around 1600 BCE.

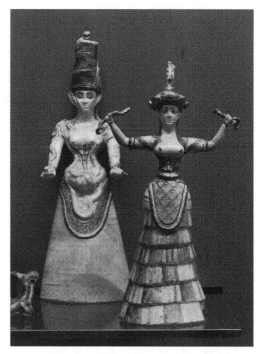

The Minoan Snake Goddesses on show at The Heraklion Museum.

A third made of ivory does exist, but common thought is it may be a forgery.

There is a belief that the more famous of the two, with the snakes in her hands, bears the possibility of having been incorrectly built, although, it is impossible to know.

Made of faience, the statue was not found in the way we see it. Its arms were missing, as was the hat and the cat on the top. That sentence suggests that the pieces were always destined to be together; that they were originally all part of one statue. However, the only reason they are, is because they fit together like a jigsaw, that the cat seemed to slot into a hole in the hat, which in turn, seemed to fit on the figure's head. From that then, we must keep an open mind as to whether Evans was right that the cat and hat were always part of her attire.

The snake goddess is fascinating, because as previously stated, a Melissa priestess works with three energies, bee, snake, and spider.

Evans surmised that she was the goddess with the other depicting a sacred servant, but I don't know. It's her sister I find more interesting since she wears the tower that features so prominently in Venus symbolism, in particular, the Phoenician Goddess, Astarte.

As previously noted in our quest to decide if Aphrodite's priestesses were Melissae: *The name "Astarte" also dubs her Cybele or Rhea. In Ovid's work* Opera *he calls Her, "the tower-bearing Goddess" that "made (towers) in cities."*[57]

Reminding ourselves that the name "Asht-tart" means "The woman that made towers",[58] the tower is the sign of the Mylitta line that would come to bear Aphrodite. This is the same lineage as the Whores of Babylon.

At Eryx, Aphrodite's priestesses were called Melissae, and as we have seen, the Eryx sanctuary was dedicated to the divine feminine long before. Perhaps connectedly, Eryx is also the name of a specific non-venomous snake genus of sand boas.

If I had to guess what species of snake she wears, I'd say a boa or python. The Oracles, Melissa Delphis, were called Pythia, and were said to breathe prophecy from Apollo, who had slain Python, and Delphyne had been the snake Goddess who had delivered prophecy there before.

Arthur Evans was fascinated by the labrys, the double axe, because, he said, there were priests at Delphi called *Labryades*. I suppose it's not without the realms of possibility that this *could be* Python. It seems as good a name as any for her. Personally though, I quite like to imagine she might be Delphyne, and that the tower we see on her head may have developed to be the omphalos that the oracle sat over at Delphi.

It's not just the one snake slithering around her. Look closely and you can discern two, just like the two serpents on the

Caduceus and indeed in an important meditation used in bee shamanism called The Serpent Flight of the Honey Bee.

This complex set of visualisations is a powerful journeying tool described in *The Sacred Sex Rites of Ishtar* by Annie Dieu-Le-Veut. She quotes from teachings by Simon Buxton:

> *We explore this knowing, specifically drawing upon the rich body of teachings from the Path of Pollen, the shamanistic tradition which works with the honey-bee and the hive in an alchemical-sexual formula, known as The Serpent Flight of The Honeybee. Within this tradition, women and men are considered to be of equal metaphysical status, with the emphasis on co-empowerment rather than co-dependency.*
>
> *The Grail – The Chalice – The Creatrix – The Hive – The Flower – The Life Givers and Life Bringers: Woman is seen as a bodily manifestation of all of these things and within this tradition she identifies with specific divine female role models, through which is awakened her innate divinity; free from shame and fear, fully empowered and openly rejoicing in their femaleness.*[70]

I wonder if the second serpent might be a viper, or asp. *Viperus berus*, the common viper or asp is venomous, but its bites are seldom fatal. It is ovoviviparous. In other words, its young mature within their eggs before their mother lays them. Hence, the young are already old enough to be born as soon as eggs are laid. In effect, like birds and bees, they too have two births. They breed every two to three years and tend to give birth in late summer to autumn, around the time of the harvest.

To outline the many surface level meanings of snake totems would be impossible. I remember being told there were 300 different interpretations, which would seem close if not accurate to me. Importantly though, there are equally as many shadow interpretations as light ones. Almost universally though, the snake is associated with knowledge, particularly that which is arcane, and with creative sexual energy.

Three specific things may be of interest. First, they shed their skins in order to grow. As they are about to do so, their eyes glaze over as if in trance. The next is they perceive their environment through scent but also through vibrations they feel in their bodies. Earthquakes for instance are often perceived by snakes before any other creature, a skill that would be useful on Crete. The third is entirely fanciful, but I recently read a story of an English lady whose snake had started acting erratically, getting on her tummy, refusing to budge, and becoming aggressive with everyone around them. The woman suspected the snake might be trying to tell her she was pregnant, and when she took a test, she found that despite the couple having given up trying, because they had had so many disappointments in the past, the test was indeed positive. Her snake, too, was a boa constrictor (although she had two of them and the other didn't do the same). That the snake is balled over the Tower Goddess' belly is fascinating too.

If the constrictor on the statuette were to tighten, the priestess would doubtless experience contractions. Indeed, one of the things that *Melissa officinalis* herb is indicated for is afterpains, as the uterus contracts back down after delivery.

Bizarrely, as an aside, if the Internet is ever to be believed, women giving birth to snakes is also a thing. There are several stories from Nigeria, Ethiopia, and India, however, arguably the most distressing, in my opinion, is that of Nalongo Nvannungi, a Ugandan woman who had given birth to twins in 2008, after her husband had died during her pregnancy. The first child was a healthy human girl, who was immediately followed by a python.[72]

The labour progressed quickly and so she birthed at home with only her sister as witness to the strange event. The python grew to be humungous, with the locals afraid of the creature. The authorities sought legal action to take it away, but Nvannungi protested that since the snake needed her to feed him 40 eggs a day, she worried he would not be able to fend for himself without his mother's care.

The trail then went dead. Periodically, I confess, I worried about the poor woman and her snake child on a continent where women have so few rights. Funnily enough, my stomach did ball up in knots when I thought about it, and it gladdened me to subsequently discover that Uganda is one of Africa's most progressive lands with regards to feminism. Over the months, I kept searching, trying to pick up the thread, fervently hoping she had not been forced to give up her child. A Liberian news agency picked up the story again in May 2020 and I was relieved to learn that, although her family had sadly disowned her, she has been allowed to keep the 30ft snake. The reporter explained that Nalongo was the name awarded to her by her tribe. It means mother of twins.[73] The respect they rewarded her made me weep. I had no-one to explain my feelings about it to, so I went and told the bees. I think they will have enjoyed it.

It's such a strange story. I wonder if it *can* be true. Could she really have given birth to a snake?

The Silent One reminded me that men's tales are full of blokes having surgery after creatures have found their way into their glans. They've then grown blocking their urethras' openings. I suppose something similar could happen to women.

Perhaps it's pertinent we cannot see where the Tower Goddess' second snake begins, perchance her skirt retains the modesty of that secret. I suppose it's not without the realms of possibility one could slither inside your vagina, especially from a river, and most certainly if you were already in an ecstatic state. In another lifetime, when female capabilities were treated with more reverence, it is conceivable the woman who was believed to have birthed a snake might have been worshipped as a Goddess.

Maybe that's who the Snake Goddess is? That thought makes me even sadder that Nvannungi was ever told she must give up her python.

Chthonic creative energy bursts out of the top of the Tower Goddess as if she has been able to control kundalini so succinctly that she is now capable of snaking through boundaries to the rest of the cosmos. Interestingly, like bees, snakes are also capable of parthenogenic birth, and will do so if they are kept in isolation. Where worker bees can only lay parthenogenic males, the copperhead snake generates females. (Whether that's their only capability is so far unclear, but researchers have never found a parthenogenetically born male as yet.)

The aprons the goddesses wear fascinate me. What debris, I wonder, were they designed to catch? Metal polish for all the gold that glistens around them, maybe. Filth from animals they have domesticated perhaps, sticky honey, or gore from sacrifices, from midwifery or funerary rituals for the dead.

When I told the hive I'd like help understanding the statues, I experienced yet another surreal Melissa moment. A gust of wind whipped round, and I became aware of washing billowing on next door's line. Their intimidatingly white sheets caught the air like glorious galleon sails, and I marvelled how some people manage to keep bed linen so clean. No muddy dogs or menstruation in that bed, I thought, and headed back into my empty house thinking once again about the dreams I'd been having of priestesses wearing bedsheets as aprons, then tearing them for poultices, compresses, using them to catch swarms...

The Silent One had temporarily left me, to make his own journey into the realm of the dead. He and his brother had navigated COVID restrictions and curfews to be with their mother, in France, and to say their goodbyes to their beloved dad one last time.

His absence overwhelmed me.

Our love is a quiet one. We rarely feel the need to even speak to one another, but he's a big man, who always smells deliciously of conifer deodorants and freshly-sawn wood. His very presence oozes from every pore of our home. I'm no good alone, and I missed his cedarwood personality, the sound of him breathing and that warm scent. The silence suffocated me, and since there was little else but reruns on the television, I decided to search for something ancient Greek to occupy my mind.

I found an old series of *A Greek Odyssey with Bettany Hughes*.

From that moment, my loneliness was transformed. I was drawn yet deeper into Greece, this time with sumptuous pictures and a very real sense of the terrifying power of their seas.

In the third episode, after being caught in dreadful storms, the beautiful Bettany's boat moored on the island of Naxos, just as Theseus' had done thousands of years before, after he killed the dreadful Minotaur.

Ariadne had given Theseus the thread that would lead him safely out of the labyrinth, in return for his promise to take her away from the island and make her his wife. He'd been true to his agreement and had set sail with her aboard his ship, but then Athena appeared to him, in a dream, convincing him to throw his fiancée overboard. So, as he approached Naxos, that's exactly what he did. Naxos was the home of Dionysos. There, his Maenads conducted ferocious inebriated rituals to ensure the annual resurrection of the god of chaos. Rescuing Ariadne from the water they invited her to join them in their ecstatic revels.

Stripped of her family connections, all clothes lost at sea, it's easy to see they might have few qualms about sacrificing her to raise their Lord from the dead.

Here, then, on my TV screen was Naxos... and very, very, *very* oddly, was a ritual to Dionysos taking place in the streets, large as life as part of 21st century festivities. Revellers were cross-dressed or wearing goat masks and bells, and the guy who was being interviewed was wearing a beautiful embroidered white apron which he revealed should traditionally have been a bedsheet, just as I'd seen them wearing in my dreams.

But why, I contemplated, were men dressed as women, wearing aprons?

The word apron boasts more than one meaning.

Not just a protective garment, the apron is also part of a ship. It's an integral component whose job it is to connect the stem to the keel, which is the structural backbone of the vessel.

Stem is also very clearly two things – part of a plant – doesn't need to be elucidated – but the keel is two things too. It's the name of the bone that means a bird can fly. It's its breastbone that connects to the wings, and then what the bird further requires, is the tendon called the supracoracoideus. That stretches up the bone of the wing, and hooks around the scapula. The sternum, to which it connects, is called the coracoid. If you trace the line of that tendon, it's very similar to how the snake seems to move around her torso.

This is made even more interesting by how Theseus' vessel – the so-called *Theoretical Ship* — is portrayed on an ancient vase called the *Francois Krater* that is now housed in the Museum of Florence, dates to 570 BCE and depicts the death of Achilles. The stern of Theseus' ship has a post called the *aphlaston*. The *aphlaston* is shaped to show two swans' heads navigating the ship. Swans are Aphrodite symbols.

The prow of the boat isn't shown on the picture, so I am not really sure how scholars know this, but that was carved into the head of a boar. The prow is the stem of the boat, the bow.

So then, if we extend that idea back to the more famous Snake Goddess, we can see that her breasts reveal the outline of her thorax – the part of the bee that allows it to fly. Her waspish waist also seems to be bound by a snake.

Seen together, the Tower Statuette appears to speak to the corporeal kundalini of the snake, but her sister seems to drag serpents from esoteric places, maybe as she draws the pneuma of Apollo from Delphyne, or even helping the snake mistress to shed her skin.

Seemingly, she, like Persephone (whom Kerényi says is Ariadne), may be psychopomp, able to conduct soul retrieval through the consciousness of the snake.

Perhaps we should consider the apron as being attached to her chest imagery, her breasts drawing the outline of the sacred lemniscate, the bees' figure of eight. The Goddess providing her endless bounty of milk and honey, or I guess, maybe, royal jelly.

Consider too, how the Melissa becomes mistress of her necktary, able to drip breast milk as evidence of ichor running through her and her newfound goddess status. After all, this is the home of Amalthea, the goat goddess, and the Melissae who were said to have fed the concealed child, Zeus, with honey.

The statues make me think of the Maenads and the sinister Sirens, the winged bird women who called out to Odysseus from Dionysos' homeland of Naxos. Keepers of the snake knowledge of kundalini, who knew how to drive it through the body to activate their necktaries, and if they were consummate, how to use it to fill their nests.

The patterns on the more famous statue's checked woollen skirt do bring a particular flying insect to mind, although, it isn't a bee.

To me, it looks like the markings of a European Flesh Fly – *Sarcophaga carnaria*.

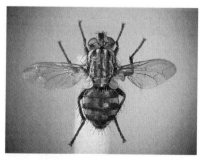

Sarcophaga carnaria – the European Flesh Fly. Photograph by Stephen Falk.

Usually found feasting on carrion, the adults live on rotting flesh although their larvae feast on earthworms. They also eat caterpillar pests and protect orchards and forested areas.

These flies, just like the shamanic symbols of vultures in the old religions, strip the flesh from the corpse so the soul can be dispatched to the afterlife.

In the original myth from the *Georgics*, Aristaeus sacrificed heifers and bulls. After nine days, bees flew out of the beasts' carcasses. Nine days after momma *Sarcophaga carnaria* lays eggs (on day 10) baby flies hatch, take to the wing, and emerge from the carrion they have been laid into.

The Snake Goddess' skirt then speaks to sarcophagus funerary practices and intervention with life after death. As such she is the Melissa – psychopomp bee who brings new souls and processes the souls of the dead.

Chapter 19

Thesmophoria

It seemed to me if I were to understand what a Melissa was, I needed to try and comprehend her belief system and get a feel for her festivals. That would seem to be a fairly simple objective, but oh the arrogance and the naivete!

It's about as easy as knitting soup!

Before we enter though, I'd like to express a word of caution and urge you to attempt to apprehend the rituals in the womb space, if you can. When you look closely enough to think you might perceive some of the elements of what they were doing, they are so clever, you either sit staring agape, or start laughing aloud. Every couple of minutes or so I have to centre myself and focus on the deep spiritual significance these multilayered rituals had. Please do me the favour of occasionally checking in with yourself to appreciate the marvellous devotion these women showed in gathering the intel to help them to merge with the Bee Goddess and her workers. I am worried that it will be all too easy, now I have written it down, to just absorb the data as facts, but these have so much more truth than just simple information.

To be clear, I have never laughed once *at* the religion, but a thousand times *with* it. Be reminded, a shaman does enjoy a laugh, but he laughs because he *knows*. For a while I felt terrible for chuckling, because, when all said and done these are religious teachings, but after a while, I just learnt to lean into the sheer brilliance and charisma of Melissa medicine.

Enjoy it.

Glimpsing the intricacies that they used to become bees is quite the most joyful thing.

Again, of course, we'll never know for certain what these things were. These are simply my observations from studying the history and the modern-day practices. Just as easily as if these conclusions are right, they could be wrong, and I certainly would not want to offend anyone's existing belief systems in the process.

As we have seen, the term Melissa had many meanings, but history is specific, Melissae were participants of Demeter's festival, Thesmophoria. It is undoubtedly the strangest, containing a ritual where they dug up a rotting pig.

Thesmophoria took place on the 11th, 12th, and 13th of Pyanopsion, in the autumn. Pyanopsion was what we would call October/November, and its first day was the new moon, so these are the three days that led to the full moon that we now know as the Hunter's moon, and it is believed to have been a fertility ritual.

The rocky terrain and soil conditions in ancient Greece would have made farming fairly arduous, and it is estimated only about 20% of the land would have been usable for growing crops. The main ones are thought to have been barley, olives, and grapes. Barley and wheat were planted in October, to be harvested in April or May. Grapes were harvested in September and olives from November through to February. Thus, Thesmophoria took place just after the honey harvest, as calves were being weaned from their mothers and moved into sheds. Ewes were being sheared round their nether regions to prepare them for mating and perhaps most pertinently grain was being sown deep into the still warm Earth, deep enough to be beneath any weeds that steal nitrogen and to protect them from scavenging birds. Indeed, Hesiod described how sowing took place as the Pleiades set in November.

These days, temperatures in Athens are around 18 degrees Celsius in November. Bees would be slowing down and getting ready to cluster inside for the winter.

I came to learn that Thesmophoria was conjoined with several festivals but particularly one called Skira.

Skira

Skira took place in the last month of the Athenian year, Skiraphorion, which was marked by the final harvest of the grain. Skiraphorion was also the month of the Arrephoria, the festival where the little girls carry the basket from Athena to Aphrodite on the Acropolis, and The Panathenaic Festival, a great celebration in offering to Athena which encompassed all manner of music and poetry celebrations and an enormous athletic competition, The Panathenaic Games.

So, this informs the first problem we encounter in trying to understand this festival. Skira is very clearly connected to Thesmophoria and is known to be one of Demeter's celebrations. Yet its timing may associate it with Athena, and because of the timing of Arrephoria, also perhaps with Aphrodite.

We know it comprised a procession led by the Priestess of Athena, with the priests of Poseidon and of The Sun.

Harpocration was a lexicographer who lived in the second century CE. By the time he attempted to make sense of the Skira, its meaning was already arcane and hidden. In his efforts, he referenced a man called Lysichides who had also previously been a grammarian, but had lived long before, having been born somewhere around 50 BCE.

Lysichides said

Skira is a festival among the Athenians from which is derived also the month Skirophorion. Those who have written much on the months and festivals at Athens, one of whom is Lysichides, say that the skira is a sunshade. When it is carried, there walk under it from the Acropolis to a place called Skiron the priestess of Athena, the priest of Poseidon and the priest of the sun. The clan of the Eteoboutadae convey it. It is a sign that one must

build houses and make shelter, as it is the best time of the year
for house-building.

See what I mean? It's all very confusing.

Skira is the name of the festival and then we're told it's a sunshade.

Get used to it. It's always this way.

Let's begin with the sunshade.

We are told it is white and was big enough to cover three people. It was held, presumably, one on each pole by four people. It was conveyed by the Eteoboutadae, which we might presume denotes them as being Priestesses of Demeter, but in fact the clan also furnished Athens with the Priestess of Athena and the Priest of Poseidon! (I told you there were no choices if you were born into that family, didn't I?!) So, we can't say for certain if our priestess is there. Nevertheless, let's carry on.

The Priest of The Sun is a strange thing, because according to *Festivals of the Athenians*, by H.W. Parke (most of the commentary on the actual rituals comes from his book, incidentally), the Greeks didn't worship a sun-god in the Archaic and Classic periods. He surmises this may mean that we are seeing a description of a later version of the ritual, which would, presumably, include Helios, or perhaps they are referring to Apollo.

I think it's safest at this point not to try and name the priest – rather to know it's somebody or some*thing* that worships the sun.

If you have lost track of the months, you are in good company, because my reference book falls open at that point now; I'll help you out. It is late May, early June, just before midsummer.

Earth is reaching the climax of her sexual energy. The animal kingdom bursts with vitality. New families of birds sing happily in the trees, lambs and kids bleat on the hills and hives are bursting at the seams. There is floral colour everywhere, but as the Mediterranean sun continues to scorch the Earth, rain is becoming less frequent too.

The month of Skiraphorion marks the end of the Athenian year which will finally end at midsummer. These last few days of the old year coincide with the time that insects are most likely to swarm. Lysichides had said this was the time for finding new homes. That is exactly what swarms are for. The colony has collected so much forage and become so successful, it has outgrown the hive and wishes to reproduce. In our case we will say bees, but the same would be true of wasps, hover flies, hornets and even ants who are also part of the same Hymenopter genus.

A large percentage of the bees leave the hive, taking the queen with them, safe in the knowledge that the workers have raised several queen cells that will be able to take their queen's place. They set off on their way, engorged, and sated with huge amounts of honey in their bellies, to find a new home. This home can be many places but is often in the canopy of a tree.

Spot the word? Skira is the name of the festival, and a canopy sunshade.

I suspect the canopy may be a bedsheet. To catch a swarm, the best way to do this is to place a sheet on the ground but leading up and into a box or skep. In simplistic terms, you shake the swarm onto the sheet and, providing you can find the queen and get her into the container, you can then rely on her to secrete pheromones that tell the others to follow, which they do in the most incredible fashion, all climbing up the sheet after her.

This "Bee March" is extraordinary. They pile into the box at tremendous speed, all clambering over each other to chase after her. Then, because some of the bees are in the air, fanning bees begin secreting Nasonov and wafting the queen pheromone about. Sticking their abdomens in the air, and fanning, they signal to their sisters that the queen is there, that everything is OK and tell them to come home.

I would suggest the priest of Helios may be a beekeeper and even if they are not actually fetching a swarm as such, they may have been re-enacting it. Historian Andrew Gough offered a similar explanation for how the priests and priestesses seem to be pulling on trees on some of the Minoan seals, just as you might pull on a branch to shake the swarm.

Sometimes there will be enough bees for there to be a second swarm too, and this is called a cast. Importantly, consider that within the next few days, at least one queen cell will hatch, hopefully mate with the drones and there will be two queens. If the swarm has cast, there will be three, which is fine as long as they can all find their own homes, because they cannot live together. Except in rare cases of supersedure, one queen will not accept another.

Remember that.

After the swarm there should be another queen, and the goddess is a queen bee.

What does that tell us? We're probably going to end up with another goddess, right? And if the colony raises more virgin queens, it could swarm and cast another, then another, maybe?

We'll see.

The festival of Skira lasted just one day and the women, we are told, observed a period of chastity, and ate large amounts of garlic. Whilst we don't find mention of the garlic in testimony about the Thesmophoria, evidence from the expense accounts from one district cites them as having bought two staters' weight of the stuff. A stater was a silver coin minted in Corinth, and it divided up into three drachmae. A drachma was about $46.50, which means they spent nearly $300 on garlic for just one festival.

According to Parke, who in turn based his theory on Lucian's descriptions of the holidays, it is most likely that the pig drawn up at Thesmophoria was likely put into the megaron (pit) at

Skira, thus symbolically investing in the next year's agricultural bounty before the old one finished.[74]

As previously said, Skira was a one-day festival in early summer. Thesmophoria took place over three days and two nights. It was the job of the *Archousai* to oversee and organise the festivals which at least, in the case of the Thesmophoria, meant making sure the women had places to camp.

At Skira, the women kneaded bread and fashioned it into the shapes of phalluses. Then, along with a pig and some models of snakes, they threw them into a pit, known as the megaron, and left them there to rot. Incidentally, pit is another of those words like nymph that has more than one meaning, doesn't it? Think about that. It might be interesting later. (Pit or stone of a fruit?)

Thesmophoria is the more researched and spoken about ritual and was celebrated right across the Hellenistic world. It is understood that just like the Mysteries, it enacted Demeter's grief of her daughter having been kidnapped.

Unlike most festivals of the polis, there were gender restrictions in place for Thesmophoria; most were mixed, except for the cult of Hercules which was restricted to men. Thesmophoria was a women-only ritual.

Let's start by thinking about the name. Earlier we met the *kanephoros* and the *arrephoros* who *"carried"* baskets. *Phoros* means "to carry".

What are they carrying here then? Thesmos means *law* or actually *ordinance*.

You thought that would help us, didn't you?

Yes, so did I. And it will, but just not yet.

Just remember though, that it means **carrying the sacred law**.

Day one of the festivities is referred to as **anhados** *(The Road Up or Ascent)*. It entailed an eight-mile walk from the Acropolis to the site. (I'm not really clear how they knew it was eight miles because no-one seems to know where the site was, but...)

Eventually, they reach Thesmophoria Land and set up camp.

On the evening of day one, *The Antlerai*, specially chosen women who were referred to as *"Balers"*, went down into the megaron to retrieve all the bits and pieces from Skira. Prior to this, the balers had been required to be ritually chaste for three days. Presumably in some kind of basket or box, they collect up partly-decomposed pig, and mouldy loaves shaped like genitalia and serpents.

Sources disagree about how much later this took place. Some say four months, others say 18 months later.

During the recovery, the priestesses made clapping noises, allegedly to scare off the snakes.

The delightfully mangy ingredients were then placed on the altar in the Thesmophoria, and then were sprinkled onto the land with seeds said to promote the fertility of the crops.

I have one resounding thought...

I really hope they didn't eat that pig.

After having read WAY too many coroner's papers to test my hypothesis that perhaps they thought the pig might help to nourish the soil, I can reveal that mouldy meat does indeed make for excellent soil improver.

This is taken from a paper written by The Corpse Project, present-day researchers interested in whether we might be better using human cadavers to nourish the planet. Fortuitously, their experiments included pigs because, apparently, they act very much like human corpses.

one year after a pig carcass (often used in research instead of a human body) has been put on the soil surface, significant increases in nitrogen and phosphates can be found in the soil underneath, but not after three years.

So, if that was what they thought, they were right. It does.

But it is really vile.

A layer for the beekeepers.

A bee disease had been my original route into what might have been taking place in lots of these rituals. It turns out, that even though doing a beekeeping course over zoom is less than ideal, it does have some advantages. When someone says that if you are unlucky enough for your hive to catch *European Foul Brood* (EFB) you have to dig a pit, your mind jumps to attention.

The attentive beekeeper might notice EFB in late spring, early summer – time of Skira – when some of the larvae seem to be all twisted up in their cells. They make unnatural C-shapes and stick along the sides or to the bottoms of their cells. Their tracheas protrude and they look silvery, almost like cooked onions; sometimes you can even see the gut through the opaque body tissue. The infected larvae first yellow up, then darken to brown until, horribly, they dry down to nothing more than rubbery scales stuck to the cells.

Now, there is another, less prevalent disease called *American Foul Brood* (named after the people who "discovered" the disease, rather than where they appeared – in this case in Australia). In AFB, it goes horribly like sticky glue, and you can kind of "rope them out" with a matchstick, but these EFB scales are dried, so the worker bees can easily remove them, which sounds like a good thing, but it also makes the disease more difficult to spot. If the infection is really bad, the colony takes on this foul, horrible fishy odour (thus the name "foul brood").

Foul Broods are reportable diseases and so the bee man has to come and have a look and do some counting. Based on how many infected cells there are in a small area, he can determine how bad the spread is and how detrimental it might become.

The counting here is key.

Armed with that data, he can predict the future of the hive.

If the number is bad, then he will suggest sacrificing the brood. You can either treat with antibiotics or a better way to treat them might be to do what's called a *shook brood*.

Carefully putting the bees onto a new frame (with a shooing action) you then dig a pit for the old one and burn it.

But here is the really strange thing: the bacterial pathogen that causes European Foul Brood is called *Melissococcus plutonius*, which is weird anyway because Pluto is the Roman name for Hades, so that's almost like Persephone's married name, but the disease wasn't named until 1970.

To have the best chance for a hive to get through the winter, it needs to have strong disease resistance, plenty of healthy bees, a robust laying queen and good winter reserves.

Having too many bees, though, can almost be as bad as having too few. The colony risks becoming cramped and it's past the ideal time to swarm. If they swarmed now, they wouldn't have long enough to establish before the cold.

So, let's look at what the bees do first.

Actually, they have already done it by now.

They kick any remaining drones out of the hive, so they don't have to feed them over winter. (No men at Thesmophoria either, remember. Actually, some literature enacts how aggressively they chased them away.)

Only female bees overwinter, and by natural wastage (remember summer worker bees only live about six or seven weeks) the size of the colony drops quickly. At peak it had grown to around 60,000 bees, but now, they are far fewer, around about 10,000 bees, but these ones are different. They must live for about six months to get the hive through the winter.

To best help them do that, the beekeeper might merge two smaller colonies. I think this is what we are seeing here – a symbolic merging of the hive.

Clearly you can't just put two loads of females together, because we are territorial creatures; the beekeeper does that by sacrificing a queen.

When a modern beekeeper merges two colonies, they place one box on top of another with a piece of paper between the boxes to separate them. The bees have such keen senses of smell that they start to nibble their way through the paper until, eventually, the pheromones of the colonies mingle, they get a feel for each other, and to all intents and purposes they unite the hive themselves.

In beekeeping these counts are vital for taking care of the colony, and I think we should consider that what works for the hive will always be echoed in the polis.

Thesmophoria was the perfect opportunity for the priestess of Demeter to perform a kind of oracular census. Not specifically about what was happening now, but what was *going* to happen with regards to births, deaths, work, and disease. It served as an opportunity to keep tabs on the numbers of youths who were getting close enough to the age where they would become mandated voting citizens, which in turn would reflect on recruitment for their military and how many potential extra mouths they might have to provide for.

The count is instrumental information for everything about the polis from education and welfare budgetary spend to how much room needs to be designated for burial spots.

With so many women in one place, there would be loads of gossip, chatter about hormones, menopause, kids... all of that info ends up in one space. Right in the hands of the priestess who takes care of the polis.

The ritual was an unparalleled opportunity to gain an extraordinary amount of data, and since there was a ritual ban on intercourse during this ovulatory period, as long as you knew who was already pregnant in the ranks, to all intents and purposes, this starts from a zero count this month again too.

Thesmophoria Day 2 was known as *Nestaia*. The "Fast".

The ritual on this day is sombre.

The women enact the days where Demeter, beside herself, would not sit upon a chair, and they sit on the ground upon leaves from the Lygos Tree. Some sources say the women slept on beds made of the Lygos. (There seem to be two opinions as to what Lygos was. Some say willow, others *Vitex agnus castus*, which we describe as Chasteberry.)

Some modern authorities, presumably trying to consolidate different narratives, erroneously describe vitex as *being* a kind of willow but Vitex belongs to the family Lamiaceae, where willow is Salicaceae. Definitely not the same botanical, so thus, we need to pick one. Willow has limited functions, and since Vitex still grows outside the Temple of Ephesus where the chaste priestesses were devotees of Artemis, I'm going to plump for that one.

Now, one of the few writers who does have the courage to write about the sacred festival is Aristophanes, but of course he can do that because, as ever, he is feeding us funny lines, taking the mick. There are clues, but again, they are witty, perhaps illuminating but most certainly obtuse.

Ashley Clements says in his paper on Aristophanes' *Thesmophoriazusae* that there is a sense that one of the characters is being guided somewhere by the other. The play opens with one character really moaning about being weary from the travel. We discover this character to be Euripides, who is lagging behind his friend. He moans...

O Zeus, will the swallow ever appear?
This man will be the death of me, tramping around in circles since dawn.

The first line makes me laugh. Does he crave the coming of spring? Is he starving hungry, desperate to swallow a morsel, because they are fasting, or is it a very rude allusion to oral sex that goes on and on?

But Clements reveals the physical comedy taking place.

Led by Euripides, who is endlessly turning back on himself, the two travellers are cross-cutting the orchestra floor in circles like cattle moving in circles of eight around the threshing room floor and have been doing so since dawn.

Interesting.

The figure of eight. The waggle dance in the beehive. Aristophanes is almost certainly making people laugh by alluding to something that the women enact at Thesmophoria. One joke is the women are played by men dressed up, but to me, that sounds like *The Walk of Infinite Flight*, re-enacting the Bee Goddess' pacing as they portray searching for The Queen of The Underworld.

Walking round is a very embodied thing in its own right. We pace when we're stressed, don't we? When we think things out. We pace when we're in pain and it's by far the most effective way of descending an unborn child into the birth canal. Gravity speeds the delivery.

All of this is embodying some kind of challenge in the body. This pacing is really a feature of when we don't know what to do next, isn't it? Accompanied, often, with wringing of the hands, back and forth, back and forth...

Oddly though, when you feel stressed and don't know what to do next, it often expresses itself in the body like Demeter's famine. It feels like hunger. Think about how much you have eaten in lockdown. You either feel like you can't face food or raid the biscuit barrel.

Or maybe you don't. Perhaps that's the point because what happens next is also interesting.

Let me ask you... if you fasted for a day, how would *you* be emotionally?

Many of you would be fine, but if I don't eat for, say, every 20 minutes or so, I want to rip someone's head off and bizarrely that's kind of what they do.

They spend a portion of the day insulting each other, shouting, and even hitting each other with some kind of plaited bark called a *morotton*, presumably re-enacting Iambe's attempts to cheer Demeter, but also as a tremendous way to get all those things you have been wanting to say off your chest.

I wonder though, are we removing the queen?

Combining two hives means one of the queens will have to die so a violent stinging battle ensues.

Let's see if we can work the medicine.

The women sit quietly on the floor and have green lygos leaves beneath them. Agreed?

That they sit meditating seems certain, I guess, but is there more that could be construed from that? I suspect they may be *Earth Sipping*, a kind of meditation that draws chthonic energy up from the ground into the womb.

In the silence, they contemplate Demeter's loss.

Vitex agnus castus affects both human oestrogen and progesterone levels,[75] which in theory could start pregnancy, I guess. Certainly, the effects of vitex are similar to *M. officinalis* in that it helps regulate menstruation and combats dysmenorrhoea.

That the entirety of the Athenian female contingent communally sit on leaves, coming up to the full moon is fascinating. Common opinion says they were doing this to align their cycles and to keep them chaste, which makes sense from a historical perspective, but from a plant healing one makes absolutely none at all.

Just sitting on a leaf, on the grass wouldn't have that effect. If they were sitting on bowls with leaves and warm water – i.e., they were steaming – that *would* make sense because the vapours would release chemicals, but the sources are clear: the women were sitting on the leaves, which were on the ground.

The leaves can only be symbolic.

So, what else can we construe from the Melissa priestess sitting on the foliage of a Chasteberry tree? (Apart from the fact that bees do love sunning themselves on vitex, of course.)

I wonder if it's not the tree itself that's important, but merely that they sit on greenery.

In pregnancy, if a woman has green discharge with a foul odour, it might herald imminent miscarriage. **A mother could lose her child.** In a "normal state" it can signal trichomoniasis – another fishy smell thing. Not at all funny, it hurts to wee or have sex and is heinously itchy. Gonorrhoea also has a discharge that can present as green.

I guess we should also consider, if there is a green discharge, she *shouldn't* be having sex. That's a thing too, right? These conditions are spread through sex.

So, what's strange, is that on one hand we hear the leaves signify that the ladies were chaste, but the picture the imagery paints would suggest that perhaps they were not.

If she is chaste, but simultaneously not chaste, how could that be?

How about if she is a married woman who is not having sex at the moment?

Maybe she has just had a baby and doesn't feel up to it yet?

In my opinion, Chasteberry wouldn't reduce libido as much as something like marjoram would for example, but it certainly would diminish it.

Certainly, if she has had a baby, she is now considered impure.

She needs to be purified. That's an interesting thing, because steams and fumigations were very much a part of Grecian and more Middle Eastern medicines. I'd fumigate with myrrh to prevent infection and close down the womb, but I guess lygos leaves would work too. Melissa leaves certainly would and are one of the foremost treatments in post-natal medicine, as well as for depression, which definitely puts you off both sex and food.

We've probably missed one of the most vital bits of the Melissa medicine there. What's the main reason you keep things quiet? Poor Demeter is rung out, we should let her sleep.

Insomnia again... a wonderful bit of healing provided by *M. officinalis*.

During the second day we hear that the women are somehow released from chains, and thus are released from confinement.

Interestingly, law court proceedings were suspended for the period of the Thesmophoria, as they were again, for the Eleusinian Mysteries. If women may have been contemplating pregnancy or illness, or indeed being momentarily released from the confinement of their homes, it is fascinating to see it aligns with other festivals of Demeter where the sacred laws seem not to apply.

I perceive two bee threads that would play out as fascinating tales.

They're complex, so let's take it slow.

That this festival takes place in October might indicate that the Melissae symbolise the winter bees that will live longer to see the hive through the colder months, so therefore are crone equivalents. Oddly, at one point two years after my last period, I started bleeding again. Biopsies and camera investigations revealed nothing. I credit the youthful change to Melissa, as much as my hair that has gone grey but chaotically lustrous.

These women sit on lygos leaves. The reason I personally love vitex so much is because, after just a week of putting two drops of *vitex agnus castus* oil in the bath about four years ago, my menopausal symptoms subsided. Specifically, my hot flushes disappeared, and I stopped suffering from night sweats.

Maintaining a normal temperature is also important in the hive.

As the temperature outside drops below 14 degrees Celsius (58 degrees Fahrenheit), bees head inside for the winter, clustering to keep warm. If there's brood, they need to maintain around 93 degrees Fahrenheit. In the winter, after all the young have gone, the core temperature drops a little, but needs to be sustained at around 85 degrees Fahrenheit to conserve honey stores.

Worker bees vibrate their wing muscles giving off heat. Bees on the outermost parts of the cluster get so cold they become motionless or can even appear to be dead. It's not yet understood how, but the bees then circulate, gradually moving the infirm to the warmth of the hive centre to revive them and then taking their place in the cold. (Think about all the myths where someone's replaced a loved one in the underworld. This perhaps also informs the Melissa's soul retrieval work and her ability to move in and out of other realms at will.)

Over time, the cluster moves toward the honey; if there is too little food, or the cluster is too small to maintain the heat of the hive, the colony will not survive the winter. Thus, most beekeepers will supplement the bees' diet with sugar syrup or pollen supplement during this time.

OK, ready for the second thread?

I think this is the secret of Thesmophoria.

Let's start again.

The women are sitting and lying on lygos leaves.

The leaves tell us they are chaste. The chaste priestesses belong to Artemis. Worker bees of course are chaste too.

In the human paradigm, given the date of the ritual, they should be ovulating, but a worker bee is sterile.

Thesmophoria is presided over by Demeter, who is mother to Persephone, and indeed the women search for her, and sit in silence because their queen is nowhere to be found.

Remember, if a hive is not queenright, the lack of queen pheromone will cause the bees' ovaries to kick in. Despite being virgins, they begin to miraculously lay young in the form of unfertilised eggs.

From either cult, Demeter Kore or Artemis', these are worker bees, and the secret of Thesmophoria is perhaps the greatest of the Melissae priestesses, the reason why the initiates of Thesmophoria were the most revered of all the Melissae.

The most accomplished priestesses in all of the ancient world, those who had fully controlled their necktary in order that they could secrete at will.

These are the **laying workers**. The unmated bees that can reproduce.

Brimo of the Eleusinian Mysteries. The Great Goddess who bore a son. Sons born forth from virgins.

This also perhaps makes sense of the symbolism for the previous day. The priestesses clapped to drive snakes away from the pig. Potentially, if the pig were a vagina, then did the snakes symbolise sperm? Were these priestesses able to control their necktaries and decide if the sperm met their egg?

The name of the third day, *Kalligenia*, meant "bearing of fair offspring". Apart from the fact there were two secret sacrifices, we know frustratingly little about this day. Hesychius is the only person who says anything about it; he says it is called *zemia* and describes a sacrifice made [to pay or compensate] for things that happened during Thesmophoria.

Deubner suggests it may have been a kind of sacrifice to pay for things that might have gone wrong during the festival,[76] which when you have a flail in your hand and you are belting a load of women who might have wound you up through the year, might have been a wise way to round things off.

The other secret festival was called the Chalcidian Pursuit. That is explained in legend as a sacrifice memorialising a time when the women had prayed for a victory in battle, and their enemies had fled and been pursued to Chalcid.[76]

Who knows who those enemies may have been.

Chapter 20

The Mysteries of Eleusis

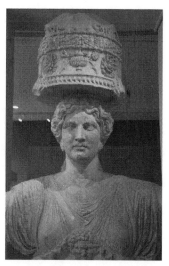

Caryatid from the Lesser Propylaea of Eleusis. C. 50 BCE.
Photograph by Carole Raddato.

My obsession with these women of the Eleusinian Mysteries pulled me under. Down and down into the womb body of the earth I fell, never wanting for a second to let the thread go.

Somehow, they called to me. I could feel these women so deeply in my being. I sensed them everywhere and saw their faces in every woman I met. I became intoxicated by them as if I too had imbibed Demeter's sacred drink, Kykeon.

The Mysteries had me in their grip.

Plutarch, on the death of their daughter, says,

because of those sacred and faithful promises given in the mysteries...
we hold it firmly for an undoubted truth that our soul is incorruptible
and immortal. Let us behave ourselves accordingly.[77]

Further, he says,

When a man dies, he is like those who are initiated into the mysteries. Our whole life is a journey by tortuous ways without outlet. At the moment of quitting it, come terrors, shuddering fear, amazement. Then a light that moves to meet you, pure meadows that receive you, songs and dances and holy apparitions.[77]

So...

For over two thousand years, in the month of Boedromian (September/October), thousands of initiates (*Mystai*) gathered at the Greek town of Eleusis, located around 20k west of Athens, to celebrate the Eleusinian Mysteries.

For a moment, feel the weight of the time that elapsed...

Two millennia.

About the same length of time that Christianity has endured thus far.

And whilst we can build a vague picture of things that may have happened, from snippets here, fragments there, all we can really get are moments of time. It's unlikely festivities remained unchanged over the years. Whilst it was important the key components remained the same, they must have evolved and developed.

Subtle changes took place from year to year. Sources we have to draw on are sparse and they give us little more than snapshots of perceptions of the cult of Demeter over time. What we discover about the Mysteries in one source, may not have remained true in a later year's celebration. As the cult of Demeter spread, it would have drawn in more local influences and then brought them back to Eleusis.

Consider that point for a moment, because I think it tells us a little something about the priestess. She'd have been measured by how efficient she was in drawing people to her festivities. One imagines she'd have wanted to integrate the latest technology, and all manner of other influences. She would have had to show great nous, her finger on the pulse and always have her ear to the ground. Continually watching what other cults were doing and then assessing how effective the changes they implemented might have been.

It's vital to remember that most of the sources that give us clues as to what the Eleusinian Mysteries might have been, were written by Christian authors. That's important for several reasons. These accounts were written centuries after the Mysteries were at the height of their fame, and the fact that they talk about it at all, when the rules explicitly state that initiates should not, suggests they are not eyewitness accounts. Propaganda maybe, hearsay probably. Conversely, perhaps we also read things that don't necessarily say they are about Eleusis, because no-one's allowed to say that, but perhaps, they highlight parts of the experience and how it changed them and their outlook on life. They tell the story of things they came to know.

That said, it's useful to consider the agenda that some of the sources may have been written in, and these particularly relate to those from the first and second centuries. The objective of these was to do the Church's bidding, to put an end to polytheism and the worship of these Pagan idols. It is safe to consider these as hostile witnesses. Accounts should be weighed for bias. Perhaps they have been deliberately made to sound outrageous and "smutty", or of course, we might find that some actually do "out" the secrets of Eleusis, because they don't consider themselves bound by its vows.

What can be used to balance this is that there were other mystery cults, whose proceedings were not protected by these same vows of silence. Parallels between things we find happening in those, when lined up against these other Christian accounts, may give us some insights into what happened.

What exactly took place in the Greater Mysteries is unclear, and is likely to remain that way, but by comparing less secretive cults than that of Demeter, by studying later sources who use the Mysteries as examples to leverage their arguments, then using dream work, I have been able to make assumptions of what may have taken place. Whether I'm right or not, it's impossible to say.

We know that The Eleusinian Mysteries were comprised of two festivals. The Lesser Mysteries, which took place in the spring, and the Greater, which were a far bigger affair, took place, in the autumn, at the time of the harvest. The festivals were to become famous the world over. For the Melissae though, they were just two of the festivals in a larger cycle that celebrated Demeter and her daughter Persephone, The Goddess of Spring. Each festival formed a vital marker that aided the construction of the agricultural Attic calendar.

The first major event of each year in the Attic Calendar then, was the Greater Mysteries in *Boedromian* which begins on the third new moon after the summer solstice, so September-October, although at the time of writing (2019) this fell on August 30th this year.

The Greater Mysteries - *13th-23rd Boedromian* - September-October
Proerosia - *9th Pyanopsion* - October-November
Stenia - *9th Pyanopsion* - October-November
Thesmophoria - *11th-13th Pyanopsion* - October-November
Halo - *26th Poseideon* - December-January
The Lesser Mysteries - *20th-26th Anthesterion* - February-March
Skiraphoria - *12th Skirophorion* - June-July

The Greater Mysteries took place every five years, then later (sometime, we hear, before the time of Herodotus) their regularity was increased, to take place annually. A prerequisite of being initiated into the Greater Mysteries was that a person had to already have taken part in the Lesser Mysteries, which took place in the spring. Eighteen months elapsed between one's initiation into the Lesser Mysteries and the initiation into the Greater. You were only allowed to attend the Greater Mysteries once.

The Passion Play re-enacted Demeter's refusal to perform her holy duties as Theia, in vengeance for her daughter being stolen from her. The play itself is thought to date back to the Mycenae period (1600 BCE to 1100 BCE) and the cult of Demeter is believed to have been established around 1500 BCE.

The story honours Demeter, and worships Kore. The initiation promised to help you to develop *kharis*, or grace, with Demeter in this life, with Persephone in death, and then perhaps by extension, some degree of grace with Hades too.

It's important, in this section, that we do not confuse Hades and the underworld with the idea of the devil and Hell. The underworld is definitely not that.

That's Christian ideology. Remember, this predates that kind of thinking.

The Greeks seem not to have sensed the underworld as based upon any impure acts they had done over their lifetimes. Simply, it was a place that was *other*. What came next, certainly, but also a place they could venture to at will. The underworld could be construed as the unconscious mind and the Lower World of the shaman, implying that should the practitioner be able to perfect their skills of walking between the worlds in life, then death might not be the barrier it would seem to be.

Even though there's a huge crossover between Greek and Egyptian theology (think about how they both deemed bees to be the souls of the dead, for example), this thinking seems to directly oppose ancient Egyptian thought. The pious Egyptian believed their entire existence on the Earth to be in *preparation* for the Afterlife. For the Greeks, *mortal life* was the big event. What came after was comparatively dull and shadowy, a sense of wandering in the wilderness, we might say. I would contend that it was the myths that moved this sense of wonder from the afterlife to the "in life".

Greek stories describe souls wandering aimlessly until given sacrificial blood to drink by Dionysos. The River Lethe, the River of Forgetfulness, ran through the entirety of the underworld, forcing them to forget everyone they had loved in life. Only initiates who drank from the *fountain of Mnensis* (memory) were able to remember the lives they left behind. (Interestingly, there is much research into Lemon Balm as a possible aid for people who are sadly living with dementia.)

What seems to have taken place is a dramatic production of the myth, followed by a display of the Holy Objects (of which we know uncomfortably little) and some kind of life-changing exhibition of sound and lights.

Any more than that, we can only guess.

The agricultural context of the play might suggest one saw Persephone rise to the surface, as if she were growing, or at least coming back to the surface to herald spring, but, actually, if you think about it, that can't be right.

Remember, this is Europe, Northern hemisphere, so Persephone would be *leaving* the earth. The re-enactment is based on the *Second Homeric Poem to Demeter*, which focuses on The Goddess' **descent** into the underworld. Her relationship with the [pomegranate] seed that must be placed into the Earth might be more accurate.

To try and gain a linear commentary into the initiation, it is easier to start with spring though, so we'll leave the Greater Mysteries for a few minutes and see what we know about the Lesser ones first.

The Lesser Mysteries
These took place between 20th-26th Anthesterion (February-March) at the eighth new moon after the summer solstice. The

Lesser Mysteries weren't always part of Eleusis, but around fifth century BCE, Eleusinian officials declared them to be a prerequisite of initiation into the Greater Mysteries.

Apollodorus tells us that legend has it that they were first congregated for Heracles who, despite being a foreigner, wanted to be initiated, in order that he could complete his 12th labour, to slaughter Cerberus the multiheaded dog that guarded the underworld gates.[78]

Historian, Theodor Mommsen, thought the Lesser Mysteries may have taken place more often than commonly thought. He describes finding inscriptions that suggest, rather than it just being an annual festival, there may even have been two celebrations of the Lesser Mysteries each year.[78]

In my opinion, it helps to avoid seeing this as an initiation, in itself, but rather as the beginning of the journey that works towards it. Kind of like the idea that every journey begins with the first step, and in this case the first step being this ritual. Scholars, Bowden and Clinton, both regard this as a first stage moment too, basing their argument for it mainly on the differences between the terminology describing the participants attending.

Commentators of the Lesser Mysteries call the initiates: *mystai* which actually translates to *initiate*, but those who have gone through to the Greater Mysteries are called *epoptai*, which means *to have witnessed*.

(I didn't know that when I first heard the Melissa voices say they "had witnessed" when I meditated on the plant.)

At this stage, we are told that initiates might be coached and taught various aspects of the Lesser Mysteries by friends and neighbours who had previously gone through initiation themselves.

This really didn't make sense to me. I struggled with it for months.

How could they do that if they weren't able to talk about it?

I mused that perhaps they were being taught how to do things like drop down into the womb space to reflect intuition (not only for women, but for men too) or how to journal dreams. Maybe there were other triggers hidden in mummery, or it pertained to something else entirely.

Over time, I've come to suspect that it means that they were being taught the secrets of beekeeping and then a trigger that something new was about to take place might have been the women running onto their roofs, with their Gardens of Adonis, that Dillon proposed took place in the spring. The mourning rite is known to have not been a state festival so that feels like spontaneous help from neighbours to me.

It's impossible to know.

Let's get scholastic again, for a minute, and try to discern what they were about to learn.

In 1891, Thomas Taylor wrote in his dissertation: *The Eleusinian and Bacchic Mysteries*:

> the Lesser Mysteries signified the miseries of the soul while in subjection to the body. The Greater Mysteries obscurely intimated, by mystic and splendid visions, the felicity of the soul, both here and hereafter, when purified from the defilements of a material nature and constantly elevated to the realities of intellectual [spiritual] vision.[78]

Gosh.

Whatever that means.

He quotes Plato who does help, a bit, when he says: "The design of the Mysteries was to lead us back to the principles from which we descended, that is to a perfect enjoyment of intellectual [spiritual] good."[78]

I like Plato's better, and yes, I would agree with that. I now look at my life and my surroundings in a much lighter and simplistic way. It has put the sheer marvel of nature at the forefront of my mind and the desire to only do good, if I can.

As stated earlier, the occasion of the Lesser Mysteries was spread out over six days. For the purposes of this section though, I have written it as if all aspects of the initiation had taken place within one ritual. It is unlikely to have been this way, but it helps us to better sense the wonder than if it were presented as the fragmented parts, which are more likely to have been the truth.

Melissa, as priestess, had opened the space for the supplicant to come into communion with The Goddess. Inside, she and the priest waited for the candidate to enter. Over the next six days, each stage of the purification would bring the seeker closer to being *mystes* – that is "initiate".

As she did, the seeker took in the space, with a mixture of excitement and trepidation, I'm sure. The air rose to meet her, redolent of latent fumes of years of incenses, not yet present in this ritual, yet somehow ingrained into the thick, stone walls. Quietly, the music of the Melissa plays. Humming, piping perhaps as if birds and the ancestral drums of Ninshubur beat methodically, taking the traveller on a journey, holding vigil then to summon her back. The Aeolian harp, placed into a draught, whispers other-worldly sounds.

Silent, the initiate enters the temple, keenly aware of a different relationship with the priestess. Potentially this is a woman she already knows but now this is hallowed time. No greetings, or how-do-you-do's, merely reverence and gratitude for her willingness to mediate the space.

The priest holds out his hands, receiving the sacrificial offering she's brought as gift for Persephone. From artwork and vases, we know that sacrificial pigs were placed upon the low lying shrine called the *eschera*.

Homer helps us picture the scene with his testimony on what a sacrifice was like, albeit this one was actually given to Apollo.

In this setting, prayers would be offered to Demeter/Kore, and the pig would be blessed with barley sprinkled onto its head, reminiscent of the bee nymphs, the Thriae.

Thus, did he pray, and Apollo heard his prayer. When they had done praying and sprinkling the barley-meal, they drew back the heads of the victims and killed and flayed them. They cut out the thigh-bones, wrapped them round in two layers of fat, set some pieces of raw meat on the top of them, and then Chryses laid them on the wood fire and poured wine over them, while the young men stood near him with five-pronged spits in their hands. When the thigh-bones were burned and they had tasted the inward meats, they cut the rest up small, put the pieces upon the spits, roasted them till they were done, and drew them off: Then, when they had finished their work and the feast was ready, they ate it, and every man had his full share, so that all were satisfied. As soon as they had had enough to eat and drink, pages filled the mixing-bowl with wine and water and handed it round, after giving every man his drink-offering.[79]

As the beast is slaughtered, the priestess shrieks her cry that signals the moment of its death. Placed onto the eschera, the creature begins to warm, to roast and sizzle. The priestess takes the oinochoē and philae, and then skillfully pours the libation, slowly, deliberately and consistently first, from the jug onto the dish, representing the Earth. Then with absolute control she directs the liquid spill onto the pig, relishing every moment of foreplay with The Goddess, who then in turn is aroused, rears up in the flames and signals her ecstatic coming.

The pig roasts slowly, gently and languidly, taking its time. The meat is rich, moist and juicy. Eventually too, porcine flesh will submit to the fire's languid embrace. Tenderly, it surrenders to its own release, separating flesh from bone.

The priest offers a libation of honey, yet more evidence of the sweetness of the supplicant's desire to commune; to come into space, and to devour the very being of The Goddess. In the erotic suggestion of the sanctuary, the supplicant softens, and she too leans into the embrace, longing for the taste of Demeter, to consume her, begging her to raise her to the moment when she can plunge into the cascade of her ritual death. Longingly, both Goddess and supplicant part their lips for the libation, eating each other in consummate union just as the bee and flower hunger for each other too.

The initiate is then led down to the Ilissos River to bathe. Freezing water engulfs her. She visualises molecules entering her every pore until she too is water for a moment.

Returning to the room, she finds the incense lit. Recipes suggest the blend probably included poppies, sacred to Demeter and Persephone, to death himself, and conducive to the narcotic journey into oblivion.

Breathing the incense, she returns from the water's caress, dripping, desperate for the warmth of Eros. The aching, the stirring in her womb is almost too much to bear. She sits, breathes deeply, exquisitely hungry for the Goddess to come.

The seeker then makes *pelanoi*, small flat cakes of honey, water and oil kneaded with sacred flour, the first fruits of the Rharian Fields. Slowly and carefully, she kneads and moulds them in her hand, creating delicacies fit for a Goddess. Looking to the priestess for reassurance of their standard, she uses her left hand to make a chthonic offering onto the fire.

Then, she's led to be seated, onto a soft white ram's fleece, placed upon a stool, in memory of the chair in Metaneira's palace; the seat that Demeter herself had sat upon, bewildered, and dazed by grief.

Blindfolded then, loss of sight sharpens her senses and all that feels familiar is left behind. Cautiously she begins her descent into darkness, her mind grasping for markers of familiarity, but instead new things emerge; things she now knows and cannot possibly have seen. Each step feels more erotic, more mysterious and foreboding, closer to a place of somewhere different, of becoming a new and mysterious version; of being veiled.

Slowly, she sheds her skin.

And as she snakes into a deeper sense of sacredness, her guides begin to emerge, whispering, moving with her body, snaking their way through her tissues, and creating a lexicon of mystery and curiosity entwined.

In the darkness, hot from the fire, languid on the fleece, heady from incense, and baking in a honeyed glow, disembodied voices float in her head.

And now, ritually purified by the altar fire, the water libation and the earthy sacrifice of cake, the priest waves the winnowing sieve through their crown chakra bringing the initiate's attention to air; as she perceives a gentle breeze above her head, she notices the incense cloud shift. Perchance she senses Dionysos separate her body from her soul.

Now purified, the initiate is brought before Demeter's priestess who will mediate the rite. Seated on the *kiste*, with the basket of mysterious Holy Objects in her lap, the priestess tempts them with a snake, offering it and asking them if they would like to receive the serpent as their totem. I'm sure many of our mystai might falter for a moment before reaching out to touch, knowing this to be a crossroads from where there can be no return; wondering if this is the right thing to do, and if, in time, it might be something they will come to regret.

Let's just excuse ourselves discretely and leave them to decide privately how their ritual will end. We don't know, because if there was any more to this ceremony, it is surely hidden by the mists of time.

A couple of notes before we move on.

First of all, the initiate uses her *left* hand to make the offering.

Offerings to chthonic deities are always made using the left and the tradition of the Melissae is called the distaff or left hand path. My son will take great delight in telling you that *his* name, Dexter, means "right handed".

Its opposite form is "sinister" which means left i.e., of the other realms. Facing with North in front of us, we might also consider how left handed could also be construed as West, the place of the Evening Star. Vesperus, as the Romans called it, was the Morning Star, which rose in the East. The Greeks knew the Evening Star as Lucifer, the Bringer of Light. Both, of course, were emanations of Venus and Lucifer rises to the left.

On another note, the Mystai were purified in the Ilissos River, which is currently enjoying an interesting point in history, as we write. Over the centuries, the stream of the myths became a river, but then erosion meant that it finally became so fierce that it caved in on itself and was ultimately lost.

After the Second World War, the Greeks hastily set about rebuilding their country. Priority was to create housing and municipal space, so they decided that rather than trying to deal with the river, their best plan would be simply to pave over it. To safely achieve that, it was culverted under a tramline, which worked for a long time, but sadly, now the tunnel is in a worrying state of disintegration. Rather than repairing it, the project known as HYDRAI plans to bring what used to be Athens' second river back to the surface. Soon, the waterway, the location of many ancient rituals, including one where they celebrated the river as a god itself, will course majestically through Greece's veins again.

So that's the Lesser Mysteries, as far as we know them, and potentially, the initiate then took the following year and a half to perfect their journeying skills, and to try to lead as rightful a life as they could, taking every opportunity to honour the gods and goddesses, in readiness for the main event the following year.

The Greater Mysteries

In the first century BCE, Cicero wrote:

For among the many excellent and indeed divine institutions which your Athens has brought forth and contributed to human

*life, none, in my opinion, is better than those mysteries. For by
their means, we have been brought out of our barbarous and savage
mode of life and educated and refined to a state of civilization; and
as the rites are called "initiations," so in very truth we have learnt
from them the beginnings of life and have gained the power not
only to live happily, but also to die with a better hope.*[90]

Initially, it was said that anyone could take part in the Mysteries
as long as they did not have blood on their hands. Later, it was
amended to being that a person must be able to speak Greek to
participate. Eventually, that changed again and demanded that
all must be "pure of soul".

So, we might assume that any Greek person, who was of
honourable character and wanted to be initiated, could be.
However, in the latter half of the fourth century BCE, the orator
Demosthanes implied there might have been a separate set of
rites for initiating the poor, in a speech where he attempted
to derail a political opponent's campaign. In one of his most
famous debates, he proclaims that Aeschines surely doesn't have
what it takes to be the kind of statesman Athens would need,
because he was so often found helping his mother, Glaukothea,
in her initiations, implying there is something a bit effeminate
about him. Whether the rites Glaukothea presided over were
connected to Eleusis, or some kind of peasant version of the
Eleusinian Mysteries is unclear.

What is certain, is you would have needed to be quite wealthy
to have been able to afford to travel to Eleusis, then paid the
dignitary fees and indeed, as you'll see, you also needed your
own mystic pig and I very much doubt they came cheap.

So, on the 13th Boedromian, 3000 prospective mystai
assembled in The Agora of Athens, to hear the proclamation of
the fest.

Three thousand excited people. Others who had already been
initiated in previous years also accompanied the procession,

merely as sightseers, since you could only be initiated once. The mystai readied themselves to witness something they may have been saving for, for years.

Let's try and imagine the scene.

The festivities will not start in earnest until tomorrow, so the landlords of Agora now rub their hands in glee, as initiates head to their accommodations and presumably imbibe a wee snifter or three.

Hundreds of vendors hustle street food, and indeed in fifth century BCE Athens, we even have specially issued coins to pay officiates for goodies and souvenirs or procuring whatever pastime might take your fancy. After all, it pays to prepare for downtime in this festival which is nine days long.

A large fayre fills the square, offering the finest produce from local producers, their stalls spill over like a cornucopia of harvest riches. Some foods are absent, however, in line with the festival laws. Pomegranates, presumably for fear of upsetting Demeter. More mysteriously, eggs, apples, fish, and fowl.

Try to reconstruct the scene in your mind again, but this time pick up the threads to weave more colour into the spectacle. Take time to focus on the fragrances you perceive. Then the sounds. What about tastes? Imagine yourself wandering around the fayre. What tastes would you, as Melissa, have tasted?

Try to remember, and as you do, ask yourself, what is it you have witnessed?

Who is by your side? Who's come on the journey for the ride? Will they complete the entirety of the initiation process with you, or have they just come to keep you company in the procession?

Breathe deeply, slowly, and feel your way into your version of Melissa. Are you dressed like someone who could afford to be initiated? In fact, if your husband is with you, could you afford to initiate both? Opulent fabrics may tell you a great deal. Remember, it's all in the tightness of the weave.

What's your sense of where you might spend the night? Where is it in relation to where you're standing now at the fayre?

Have a look in your hand. There's an Eleusinian coin. Miniscule, no bigger than the size of a raisin and yet clearly marked in tiny bas relief. On one side is Triptolemos, surrounded by his corn, and on the other is a pig encircled by a wreath.

How many more have you got to spend?

Where have you stashed the rest?

Relish the pride you feel in having got this far. Not many people get to hold one of these special coins in their hands. What physical and emotional sacrifices have you had to make to earn the money to exchange for that coin?

Sense your body.

What's on your feet? Consider your shoes. Work your way up. How do your legs feel? Are you aching from being on your feet all day long, or are you still full of vigour? How does your bladder feel? What about your stomach? Do you have an awareness of where the toileting facilities would be, and how are you going to manage that with 3000 people around? To help you with that, going to the toilet in front of other people was a sign of nobility, and one would sit on a marble slab with water flowing below. One washes one's hands in flowing water too.

How are you feeling about all of this? Getting ready for what will be the highlight of your religious life… What emotions and epiphanies flutter in your stomach?

The sun sets on the first day of festivities, and most likely, our mystai is anxious and excited, but she will have learnt the importance of speaking to the goddess before she sleeps. Of calling on the Melissa priestesses and asking them to visit her in her dreams. Of asking her for insights, or protection or simply to be with her in these fundamental days of this life as she indemnifies herself for what comes next.

And as she sleeps, who knows what things she will learn, what ideas will form and what messages she might receive, but as she wakes on the 14th Boedromian, her heart feels full of anticipation of what will come next.

For today, she will see her again, the Priestess of Demeter. Full of ceremony, the priestess will escort that same basket of sacred objects the mystai had seen at the Lesser Mysteries.

And so it began; the first day of the Mysteries.

The sacred things, the hiera, were carried to Athens from Eleusis, along the *Hiera Odos*, the Sacred Way. Local villagers created an honour guard for the priestesses of Demeter and Persephone who carried baskets on their heads. Their route was clearly marked by small stones laid onto thick soil and protected from rain erosion by taller bricks edging the sides. It was pristine and cared for with love. A roadside stone still credits its upkeep as the responsibility of the Priests of Demeter and Persephone. It is dated 421 BCE.[81]

Days later, they would return to Eleusis accompanied by thousands of pilgrims. Their sacred journey was punctuated by many stops to make offerings, prayers, and libations, each sanctuary hiding its own special meaning.

As evening fell, excitement filled the air. The news that "They're here" spread like wildfire through Athens. Everyone rushed outdoors in the hope of catching a glimpse of two of Athens' most beautiful women. And with their smiles and sacredness the priestesses brought Athens good fortune and the blessings of the goddess.

The priest of Demeter ascended the steps of the rocky outcrop of the marvellous Acropolis. Out of courtesy to the Priestess of Athena, he announced the arrivals of the sacred entourage of Demeter. In his reverence, he ensured goodwill between the presiding goddesses of two regions. Then, amidst great jubilation the sacred procession followed him, through the Agora, up to the sanctuary dedicated to Demeter in Athens, the Eleusinian.

The following day, I'm sure our mystai probably awoke with some trepidation aware of the strange day that was about to unfold. She gathered up her travel companions, various foodstuffs, sacred or otherwise, and finally armed herself with a mystic pig and towel.

From the Eleusinian, the priest declared the day as *Agyrmos*, a day of ritual purification for both the pilgrims and the pigs. With that, our mystai joins the mob, heading towards the sea.

Now, I am not sure if my mind just thinks this was so bizarre it keeps going over and over it, but the more I have worked on this research, the more often I have dreamed I was there trying to remain, at least in part, decent amongst the waves, while trying to keep hold of my squirming pig.

I've had dreams of being an older woman watching someone else try to scrub and anoint their pig. Howling with laughter as the older me remembered having tried, furiously, to hold onto my own beast tightly when I had been younger too. Actually, in the dream, the old me laughed so much that she ended up having to get in the water to clean up anyway, because she'd laughed so much, she wet herself. Funnily enough the younger companion saw the funny side then.

Whether memory or imagination, I have this vivid picture of thousands of furious squealing pigs. That might have been entirely accurate, because Plutarch describes an occasion where the mayhem got so bad that a prospective initiate got eaten by a shark, presumably enticed by the water swimming with blood.

Consider though, that, amongst the screeching, the cries of the gulls, the crashing of the waves, and potentially dodging the odd jellyfish – or shark – each initiate must find a way to quieten their spirit, to come into communion with the goddess and ask her to accept her gift of the pig. If ever there was a test as to how well she'd practised her focusing skills, this was the day!

Sources are scrambled now. Many suggest that the pigs were sacrificed that evening. Others suggest two days later. After a day in the water, it must have been one heck of a feast with multitudes of very hungry people!

Procession Along The Sacred Way

Boedromian 19, and the mystai reassembled in the Agora, forming a procession to the Sanctuary of Demeter at Eleusis, to retrace the steps the priestesses had journeyed those days before.

Leading the way, the dignitaries, the priestesses, once again raised baskets onto their heads and Plutarch tells us that this time they were secured fast with a red ribbon. The Priestess of Demeter carried a single staff of myrtle (although some authorities say several sticks joined with rings).

Following the priestly sect was a cavalcade of Greeks, their donkeys laden once again with paraphernalia including torches for the ritual later in the week.

It must have been hot and dusty, but presumably that would not have fazed the crowd. Fourteen miles, the cortege covered. Every few dozen meters, they reached another sanctuary or shrine, venerating it with sacred dances, sacrifices, ritual washings, and libations. Plutarch tells how the youth of Athens, the Ephebes, ran with the procession occasionally catching someone's arm to adorn it with a brightly-coloured ribbon.

According to Aristophanes, the entire journey was accompanied by pipe playing and song. Soon, the chatter became praise, hymns became paeons, and as spirit began to consume them, the voices joined in unison to chant:

Iacch, o Iacch,
Iacch, o Iacch,
Iacch, o Iacch.

Invoking the god, Iacchos (closely related to, and often identified as Dionysos) – they urged him to appear.

Plutarch described the scene in his account of the battle of Salamis, saying:

a great light flamed out from Eleusis and an echoing cry filled the Thrassian Plain, as multitudes of men, together, conducting the mystic Iacchos in procession...

As the fervour of chanting continued, a strange twist of consciousness took place as the crowd began to taunt each other, young scorning old and poor making fun of the rich. They entered a phase of betwixt and between. Just as the handmaiden, Iambe, had poked fun of the disguised Demeter to lighten her mood, strangely and arcanely, social structures fell away. The usual constraints of society and order no longer applied; laughter with no hierarchy perceived. A level playing field for all, and as social constructs dissolved, they entered the gates of Eleusis.

I've often reflected on how it must have felt to have barrelled through those gates, bawdy, lewd and coarse. Then suddenly in front of you, you saw the Kallichoron Well. The place where a frail old woman had wept for the loss of her child.

It must have been such a sobering moment.

Kallichoron literally means "beautiful dances", and Euripides, in *Ion*, speaks of how the pilgrims danced into the sanctuary. As the long line of initiates snaked around the well, a vital part of the initiation began to take place, the circle representing cosmic order being brought to the human world.[82]

Homer's *Iliad* says:

The dance of the youths and maidens is distinctive. It is a ritual dance performed with great care, by dancers scrupulously dressed in their best garments. It is made up of a crisp, rapid, circular figure, followed by a movement of two lines in opposition to one another.

Round and round they went. Swirling and turning, as the breeze tossed their ribbons into the air creating a vibrant tableau of colour. Twisting, swirling, spinning, and as the dancers, spun so the particles of the universe and divinity crept ever closer in.

Eventually, exhausted, the twirling and laughter quietened. One by one, they lay down to sleep, and many hours after the last rays of the sun disappeared, silence descended on Eleusis. A peaceful stillness resided, as each person lay protected by the glow of several thousand torches flickering under the stars.

The sun rose and climbed high in the sky. Helios bore witness to sacrifices made by the Archon Basileus and the overseers of the festival, the *Epimelêtai*. Sources describe muscular youths hoisting a live, sacrificial bull aloft, so all could bear witness as the priest slit its throat. An impressive display of the vigour of Athenian young men; humility and devotion to the goddess.

Finally, at sunset the crowd entered the main area of the Eleusis sanctuary, the Telesterion, where the initiation would take place over two consecutive days. One by one, they washed and cleansed themselves before entering the main area.

The Telesterion building, itself, measured about 255-270m² and seated about 3000 people. Inside were five rows of pillars and Plutarch described how people jostled and shoved in a bid to secure themselves the best seats.

At the centre was the *anaktora* where the sacred objects were kept and displayed.

Plutarch recalled initiates filling eight rows of stepped seats, all seated in awestruck silence, but it was the mystic whiff of torches as they were extinguished, then waiting in the darkness for the initiation to begin, that left the biggest imprint in Aristophanes' memory.

The first part of the festivities was the passion play acted out by the highest officials. We heard earlier that the Eleusinian priesthood shook their purple cloaks at Alcibiades after he parodied the drama at a friend's dinner party. That it could be performed in a domestic setting suggests its cast was probably small.

Apollodorus describes how the initiates were then sent outdoors with their torches to look for Demeter's lost daughter. Eventually the Hierophant sounded his gong to call up Persephone, and Lactantius tells us the initiates reassembled with rejoicing and brandishing of torches.

But now, we too are in the dark, because the blanket of secrecy is complete. People have made guesses, of course, usually by drawing on things that happened in other cults.

In the second century BCE, Alexander of Abonoteichus initiated a new mystery cult he had modelled on Eleusis. His cult worshipped a snake god called Glycon, which has since been called fraudulent, but it is interesting to bear witness to elements he likely stole from Eleusis. The climax of *his* mystery took place over two nights, contained a kind of *hiero gamos*, or sacred wedding, and then, on the second night, a birth of a child.

Plutarch described how, in around 300 BCE, Ptolemy Soter invited the Eleusinian hierophant, Timotheus, to Alexandria, whereby he asked him to devise a Mysteries of Isis, as a means of growing his new cult of Serapis. Subsequently, in second century CE, these Mysteries were attended by a Cretan poet, Mesmonedes, who then wrote about what he had witnessed. He says, *Chthonios Hymenaios*, which historian Jan Bremmer feels must translate to:

Subterranean wedding
Birth of a child
Unspeakable fire
Harvest of Kronos
The showing of the sacred things

Asterius says, *"Nor does Demeter wander and bring in Celeuses and Triptolemus and snakes and perform some acts and undergo others,"* which might infer some sort of sexual act took place between

Demeter and King Celeus, but the statement is not definitive and, if there was such an encounter, it's not clear if it actually took place within the ritual.

The Christian Bishop Asterius of Amaseia in Pontus asked of his Pagan readers:

> *Are not the mysteries the core of your worship? Are the dark crypt not there and the solemn meeting of the hierophant and the priestess, the two alone together? Are not the torches extinguished while the crowd believes its salvation lies in the things done by the two in the dark?*

Burkert suggested the crypt may have meant the "gateway to the underworld" but there is no evidence the word ever meant that, and no-one has ever found an underground chamber.

There are suggestions there may have been dancing, which seems likely since bees do dance, and there was certainly speaking and singing because accounts describe the hierophant's wondrous voice. This lifelong office was held by a male Athenian citizen of advanced years, who devoting himself to the service of the temple, lived a chaste life. To observe this chastity, it was said that he would ritually anoint himself with hemlock juice, which, by its extreme coldness, was said to "extinguish in a great measure the natural heat."[83]

Plant medicine has no side effects, only many main effects. Hemlock has myriad properties including promoting impotency, or even killing you, if you use enough of it. It is also a trace ingredient of witches' flying ointments. Traditionally, the cream is rubbed onto a besom (the ritual name for a witch's broom) since the ingredients are best absorbed rectally or trans-vaginally, and the witch places it between her legs. Constituents absorb into her bloodstream manifesting hallucinations, a bodily buzzing sensation, and the sensation of flying.

An inscription from the second century CE talks about the Eleusinian *hymnagôgoi* but it is unclear whether that would have been a choral piece, or congregational singing.

The hierophant's beautiful voice might be the most enchanting allegory of all.

You might ask yourself, apart from eating honey and shagging, what is the point of drones? Common thought is their usefulness may be something to do with their deep, rich song. Something about it means the ladies are simply happier when drones are about.

In *Song of Increase*, Jacqueline Freeman tells how her bees taught her:

> *Drones are exquisitely conscious of the sense impressions within their hive. They are also fully connected to the historical context within which all bees dwell, and they transmit this knowledge to the unborn bees through their magnificent song. The drones' song tells new bees about the journey of bees throughout history, from the ancient past to the present, and how the bee kingdom moves forward into its future.*[84]

> *Their song describes the spiritual and functional purpose of honeybees in the world. When the holy drones sing to the pips, they are much like people of Aboriginal and African cultures who sing ceremonial birth songs. These tribal people understand that the birth songs welcome babies into this world and convey important knowledge, telling them where they have come from and how they and their tribe will move into the future. These tribes believe that people who are born without hearing their birth song struggle throughout their lives, because they are untethered and don't comprehend where and how they fit in the world.*[84]

> *While the drones sing their ancestral song, the babies are also surrounded by a second song, sung by the maidens: the hive's*

song. This vibratory lullaby permeates the eggs in their cells and speaks to them about life within the hive in the present moment. Bees need to know the individual tasks they will take up inside and outside the hive – the role of bees in the world. The song of the maidens tells the bees what they will do once they are born; the song of the drones tells them why they will do that. The drones are the only bees who sing the Song of Ancestral Knowledge.[84]

The drones convey to the hive's future forager maidens the intelligence they will carry out into the fields and bring to the flowers. If the maidens don't hear the drone song and don't acquire this knowledge, they will be less able to fulfill their role in the fields and on earth. In a robustly healthy hive, each bee resonates with the drone song. Inside the hive, the drones bring forth the balanced sound that vigorous hives make — the sound of healthy, exuberantly alive hives.[84]

I've marvelled at how friendly drones are myself; not having stingers, they often land on my arm as I write, staring at me with their massive eyes that stretch almost over the entirety of their heads. I'd found it creepy at first, but I love Freeman's words that the bees told her the drones were out collecting knowledge. Now, I always read the words I have written for them to take back.

Guard bees are fascinating to watch when a drone is about. My hive has an entry of three 1cm holes. On busy days, I leave three open, but as the wasp season starts, I close two of them down. The girls are quite happy to wait their turn and queue. But drones don't have to stand in line, the sisters step aside to allow them in – so they head to the brood cells, Freeman said.

It took me a while to get the hang of so many things to look for when I opened the frames; the first thing was to try to distinguish my queen, who is marked, but I was determined to learn to identify her properly. Looking for unusual abdomens inevitably means you will find drones, who are larger and have a different shape. She is right, most of the drones *are* on my brood combs, happily singing away.

I love this. It feels like it explains how drones know where to congregate to mate, and how new worker bees know what their jobs should be when they hatch.

A gnostic author describes:

Just as the hierophant [...] at Eleusis, when performing the unspeakable mysteries amid the great fire, calls out at the top of his voice...

"The revered Goddess has given birth to the sacred boy, Bromo to Brimos," that is, "The strong one has borne a child."

The announcement closely resembles a line from Euripides' work, *Supplicants*.

You too revered Goddess once gave birth to a boy.

Plutarch describes how the ritual then worked towards its climax and participants were subjected to some terrifying experience...

The soul suffers an experience similar to those who celebrate great initiations (...) Wandering astray in the beginning, tiresome walkings in circles, some frightening paths in darkness that lead nowhere; then immediately before the end all the terrible things, panic and shivering and sweat and bewilderment. And then some wonderful light comes to meet you, pure regions and meadows are there to greet you, with sounds and dances and solemn, sacred words and holy views; and there the initiate, perfect by now, set free and loose from all bondage, walks about crowned with a wreath, celebrating the festival together with the other sacred and pure people, and he looks down on the uninitiated, unpurified crowd in this world in mud and fog beneath his feet.[85]

Tertullian says they were shown a phallus. Since phallic symbols are believed to have played a prominent role in Demeter's festivals that doesn't seem unreasonable. Another Christian author relates there were "acts about which silence is observed and which truly deserve silence".

One gnostic author asked: *"What is the marvellous, most epoptic mystery there, an ear of wheat, harvested in silence."* It is thought the wheat accompanied the statue of Demeter.

Chapter 21

A Final Curtain Call from The Insects

So, there we have it, the Eleusinian Mysteries.

While I was researching, I had read the Hindu tale of The Goddess Of Black Bees. Bhramari Devi's story tells of how she recruits all the six-legged insects to overcome a terrifying demon Arunsara. I was enchanted by the bee association with the polis and wondered if perhaps there were others lurking in the myths. So, I amassed as much etymological knowledge as I could.

Soon, other insect parallels appeared. In the spirit of The Bee Mistress being the Queen of Synchronicities, I thought I would point out a few.

There are several ant connections.

The Myrmidons were fierce warriors from Thessaly who pledged their allegiance to Achilles when he led them into battle in the Trojan wars. It was believed their name came from the word *"myrmekes"* which is ancient Greek for the Myrmex species of ant.

Their origin story goes that Zeus made his son, Aeacus, king of the uninhabited island of Thessaly but then when he lost all his allies to a monstrous famine, he had no-one to help defend his kingdom. Aeacus prayed to his father while gazing at some ants one day, pleading with him to provide an army for defence. In answer, before his very eyes, Zeus transformed Thessaly's ants into men. From then on, they were called Myrmidons. Strabo said they were given the name because of the impressive way they excavated the earth, spreading soil over the rocks so they would have ground to till, and then living in dugouts, refusing to use any of it for bricks.

There was also an Attic maiden, beloved by Athena called Myrmex, who boasted she discovered the plough, when actually it was Athena. In vengeance, the goddess of wisdom turned *her* into an ant too, perhaps for imagining herself bigger and stronger than she was.

According to Philochorus, another Myrmex was also father to Melite, from whom the Attic demos of Melite derived its name. (Melite encompassed much of the real estate of the Acropolis and was also the name of a Greek settlement in Malta.)

There are other ant stories.

In the Labyrinth tales from Crete, Daedalus went missing after the death of his son, Icarus. King Minos, wanting to flush him out, set an enigmatic competition. The challenge was to pull a thread right through a conch shell.

Minos had promised an attractive incentive for the successful winner, which in turn tempted King Cocalus of Sicily, who suspected he may have a hidden advantage. A secret weapon if you will. He was actually hosting Daedalus, who was staying in his house convalescing. Knowing that Daedalus loved these kinds of puzzles and thinking it might cheer him up, he invited him to help, oblivious that this could betray his friend.

Daedalus pierced a hole in the shell tip, then smeared it with honey. He tied the thread around an ant, which then cleverly created a brilliant strategy. Drawn in by the honey's delicious sweetness the ant calmly followed the spirals of the shell, taking the thread with it. Daedalus was caught in a honey trap.

Many a hive has been ruined by an invasion of ants.

Probably unrelated, but a huge part of the imagery in my head, is that there are often games attached to sanctuaries, where competitions were offered to please the gods. The Olympic Games are an obvious example, but there were more. Delphi had the Pythian Games, and whilst Skira was taking place, there was also the huge Panathenaic Games, where it is said that young men carried vine branches.

At Eleusis, I'd imagined them being told they were all following Adonis' pig around the universe, tethered to

Aphrodite's figure of eight. Rushing up onto rooves to make his gardens, down into the water, up the side of the Acropolis again, tracing out Venus' pathway in the landscape, like this well-trained swarm of bees always serving the goddess of love.

But it seemed to me, that could only be the women's revelation, because the men weren't bees.

That created a dilemma then, because I was already sinking under research, so the last thing I wanted to do was get involved in the men's stuff. But as I looked at the rituals, something else jumped out. The men didn't just carry these vines at Panathenaea, there were olive and vine branches in several other rituals too. I imagined these ants, continually in search of honey, always pulling threads behind them.

Like bees, the ant family *Formicidae* is enormous, containing about 140 genera.

They too are eusocial, living in colonies and adhere to a hierarchical structure, run by workers.

One doesn't necessarily think of them as being part of the Hymenopter genus, but of course, in mating season hundreds of them grow wings and leave their nests to mate.

After the nuptial flight, drones die, and the queens gnaw off their own wings, then dig down into the ground to tend their colonies. They make permanent nests in soil, under rotting wood, stones, or in trees.

Coincidentally, bees suffer from their own kind of parasites, called varroa mites. Varroa can be treated using thymol or formic acid. (Or you can dowse the ley lines. Seemingly, they don't like living in hives that sit over black water channels.)

Another one of my obsessions took me to an amusing insect place too.

The most terrifying of the deities must surely be Hades.

To me, Hades seemed inextricably linked to Osiris and that was confirmed in the *Interpretatio Graeca*. The Greeks thought that too. Osiris is in part Serapis, whom the Greeks revered as Dionysos.

So, Osiris is the Egyptian Hades, is he not?

Aedes aegypti is the Latin name for the Yellow Fever Mosquito.

Mosquitoes claim more souls than any other creature on the planet, and it is often imagined that they all bite, but that's not true. It's only the females because they need so much protein to procreate. Their thirst for blood becomes problematic around September/October, and especially near water. They breed in wells. It might explain why the Eleusinian ritual seemed to mark her return, even when it was done in Autumn. While they are most famous for biting people, if Persephone were a mosquito, The Goddess would only require blood sacrifice when she was pregnant around the time of the mysteries because mosquitoes, like bees, mostly feast on nectar.

Persephone and Hades' daughter, Melinoe, is described as being the saffron-clad bringer of nightmares. Symptoms of yellow fever are high temperature and delirium, loss of appetite and a sensitivity to light. Its name refers to the jaundice that some patients develop.

Research shows the citronellol in *M. officinalis* has larvicidal, ovicidal and repellent properties against **Anopheles stephensi**, an Asian and African malaria vector,[86] and indeed there is research currently being done in Brazil to try to use micro-molecules of Lemon Balm against *Aedes aegypti* too.[87] That the priestesses seemed to smell of Melissa may have protected people from getting bitten at Eleusis and Thesmophoria.

What amused me though, there is a plant that mosquitoes hate even more. If Hades was Aedes aegypti, it was a genius stroke on Persephone's part to turn Minthe, a former lover whom she distrusted around him, into a plant. Mosquitoes cannot abide mint.

Poor Minthe was properly screwed, wasn't she?

It occurred to me that Maenads were often described as ripping their clothes, which also seems reminiscent of the feverish symptoms of malaria and how the heat may make you feel like you burn in the fires of Tartarus. Perhaps these powerful shamanesses shapeshifted into mosquitoes? If they did, then there may be a suggestion that they knew how to merge with other critters too. Indeed, the famous necklace found at Chryssolakkos Necropolis looks more like a mosquito than a bee to me.

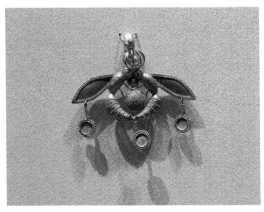

Bee pendant, gold ornament, Chryssolakkos Necropolis near Malia, 1800-1700 BCE. Photograph by ZDE.

Famously, the Egyptians buried their dead with scarabs which were believed to roll a great dung ball around the sky. You might ask yourself how these creatures, who symbolised Ra and life itself, knew which way to go. The sun maybe, or the moon? Nope, scarab beetles are the first creatures discovered to orient themselves by the Milky Way.[88]

I'm not entirely set on Persephone being a mosquito, because I also have another theory for her. I wonder if she might have been a wax moth, being "The Honeyed One". Wax moths fly at night and unlike bees *do* mate in the darkness of the hive, which would then explain the Eleusinian subterranean wedding.

Moths are attracted to torchlight which would be rather magical if you were searching for her at night, until hundreds of them arrived. Women had to sacrifice their fanciest frocks if they wore them to the temple and wax moths devour all the bees' leftover silk.

I suppose there is a very slim chance both could be right as presumably different storytellers proposed different riddles. Maybe that's why some myths prevailed while others slipped away.

I must give grateful thanks to American friends who delighted me with tales of the cicadas as they emerged this year. I'd never really heard about them before. Like the Galli, they too make their noise on their tympanum and sound like the clattering of cymbals.

In the end, I chose not to include a long chapter where I studied Ariadne's death, but I worked and reworked the myth until I eventually had an idea of what *Damnameneus* might be. The word appears in the *Ephesian grammata*, a protective spell supposedly sacred to the goddess. It means "hammer" and was the name of one of the Cretan dactyls, born when Rhea pressed her fingers into the Earth as she gave birth to Zeus.

Apart from being a soldier, Dactyl also means finger.

The *Kouretes dactyloi* were the guards recruited to watch Zeus when Rhea had given birth to him and the Melissae fed him honey.

They distracted the attentions of the murderous god, by hiding the newborn's cries with their clattering. A vitally important job because had he been discovered his father would have eaten him. It was the Death Watch.

The Death Watch Beetle likes to lay its eggs in wood, where other insects have been, but their eggs can pupate for up to ten years before they hatch. If timber is neglected and allowed to get damp, it becomes porous enough for the fully-grown adult beetle to gnaw through.

If you sawed into the wood, you might see the adult, and even the pupa, but probably not make any connection, because there is no other evidence of the baby ever having been there.

However, eventually, it will want to mate, so it tap-tap-taps on the wood, which is unbelievably irritating after a while. It's impossible to resist and you become entirely focused on the noise.

The Kouretes would seem to me to be eternally protecting the human world, disguised as Death Watch Beetles.

When I was researching Ariadne, I became rather obsessed by the Theseus tale, and I saw several other insect connections there. In the story, it says that, before he set sail home, Theseus put holes in other people's ships, but there is no explanation of how he did it or why. That bothered me. There didn't seem to be a motive at all. I dreamed of Dionysos shapeshifting, as he had whilst on a ship in one of the Hercules myths and I wondered if he had become a woodworm. That's not as random as it sounds because Theseus' ship remained famous and intact long after the hero had died, and indeed set sail each year to Delos, to continue Theseus' promise to Apollo that he would eternally give thanks for a safe return from his time with the minotaur.

Plato's *Socrates* proposed the question that if every piece of wood had now been replaced in Theseus' ship, was it, in fact, the same vessel? The question became known as the Theoretical Ship. Clearly, there is a psychological analogy based on spiritual changes the personality goes through… are we ever anything but a work in progress… but what about the wood?

Could it be woodworm?

Oddly, I found woodworm is the slang name for the young of **ambrosia** beetles!

In fact, boats don't get woodworm. They get shipworms. I wondered if the carpenter's endless battle against *Teredo navalis* might have inspired the ouroboros symbol.

I wondered if there were any insects that attacked stone. Surely not... You have no idea!!! It's a whole realm of misery for stone masons, but my favourite was a naughty little blighter that attacked *fruit* – the Date Stone Beetle.

The species uses the haplodiploid sex-determination system: while males are haploid, females are diploid. That is, males are born from unfertilised eggs, just like bees are.

Unmated females give parthenogenic birth to males, but mated females produce males and females. When scientists collected specimens from stones, roughly 90% were adult females.

Their story is extraordinary. Here's what happens.

An unfertilised female will fly around searching for a fruit tree. We'll say a date palm, but it could just as easily be a nutmeg, or cinnamon bark, a betel nut, or an almond. She buzzes around and then settles upon some fruit. She's strategic in her endeavours.

First, she nibbles through the flesh, down to the stone, halting its growth. Two or three days later, the fruit falls from the tree.

Males can't penetrate the stone, so it can only be a female that does this.

She bores into it, creating a chamber, into which she lays five or six males.

Remember, she hasn't needed any help with this because males are born from unfertilised eggs.

She waits until the first hatches. She mates with him then she disposes of his brothers by eating them, thus stacking up the protein reserves she needs.

She extends the chamber and now lays about 70 eggs. Females hatch, then mate with their brothers. It takes about three weeks for lava to pupate. Mated females live about 73 days, about ten days longer than the unmated ones.

Do you remember what they called Ishtar?

I'll regurgitate...

She was often referred to as "Lady of the Date Clusters".

Even the Date Stone Beetles' wings are fascinating! They have four. The rear two are for flying but then they have a hardened armoured front pair that protect them. Could that be the imagery of Mylitta, the honeyed, sweeter side, which can fly, and the protective warrior goddess?

One of Ishtar's earliest representations was as an incarnation of the grain storehouse; her symbol came to be the grain store gates.

Wheat is haploid too.

Whether the Eleusinian priesthood knew it was a mystical parthenogenetic birth, when they held it up at the climax of their ritual, we'll never know.

Hekate then? The goddess of witchcraft and magic. Who was she? I don't know really. Perhaps as *Phosphoros* she was a firefly? She ruled boundary places, and they do like to be on the edges of forests. Surely, everyone loves those, and she is remembered as being the most beloved.

Again, I edited out reams about Hephaestus, but poor soul, Aphrodite treated him abominably. Cheating on him, even as he could be heard tapping away making her jewellery. He seems to have been indestructible. Whatever Aphrodite did, he just kept coming back. Hammering on metal, he rattled all day long. Poor cockroach in the armoury. Gentle, resilient protective lover.

I agree with Aristophanes when he named his play *Wasps*. They must feature somewhere, but I'm not sure where.

At first, I wondered if it were the Galli, yellowjackets in their saffron coats, and maybe it was a jibe at those who only pretended to be stingless eunuchs.

Lately, I've come to think that perhaps *Dionysos* could be the wasp, coaxed away from the bees' honey stores, into wine-laden wasp traps laid by the Maenads. Also pollinators, wasps' favourite plants do seem to be the ivy that protects my garden's boundaries and snakes around the Maenads' heads, along with the pine tree and fennel symbolised by the thyrsus staff.

Who knows if I am right or wrong, but I adore the notion that it might be the most horrible bugs that protect us most.

My out and out favourite though was to discover the creature that reminded me most of Iambe.

Iambe fetched Demeter a ram's fleece stool to sit upon and then she finally managed to make her laugh when she showed her genitals.

Common thought is she may have been a hermaphrodite.

Although, I do like to think that maybe she tells us she was a Melissa when she tells her name, "I am bee". I also wanted to know if there were any hermaphroditic insects.

Ladies and gentlemen, allow me to introduce you to *Icerya purchasi*, better known as the Cottony Cushion Scale, a tiny blight on houseplants.

Originally identified in New Zealand in 1878, the scale feasts on around 90 different varieties of woody plants, most notably citrus and pittosporum species. Scales are inoffensive little things that suck on plant sap for a living. Encased in bizarre waxy shells, you probably wouldn't even recognise them as insects. To the naked eye, a cottony cushion scale looks like a dollop of shaving foam.

Under the microscope though...

I'm sorry, dude. You look like a tampon!

To say their evolutionary traits have got things sorted is an understatement. If you thought the tale of the Date Stone Beetle was the stuff Greek myths were made of, just wait till you hear this.

Mostly hermaphrodites, with the exception of the occasional pure male, almost all Cottony Cushion Scales are both male and female. Reproduction is achieved by having sex with themselves and using their own sperm to fertilise their own eggs.

Amazing right? Oh, you ain't seen nuthin' yet!

After the young have been conceived, yet more sperm invades the embryo. This "infectious tissue" then leaves sperm-producing organs inside the daughter which then eventually fertilises its eggs.

I got incredibly confused by the whole "he/she/it" pronouns issue here, so to explain that the odd few pure males look different to the standard hermaphroditic scale, which is described as being the female, in contrast to the male, and thus is described as being the "daughter".

So, scale insects are grandfather, grandmother, father, *and* mother to all of their grandchildren.[89]

Yes, Demeter. That made me laugh too!

Of everything, I wished I could come up with an answer for what the labrys is, but alas, if it is to be a plant healer who cracks that puzzle, it's not this one.

At least, not yet.

But I like to think the resemblance of the stalactite in the Dactyl cave to a termite hill might hold the key. Just as pyramids resemble ants' nests, both internally and out, I love the idea that the crunch of the axe would despatch millions of termites out into the world.

Why? Because where ants are workers, termites which are also hymenopter species are divided into "workers" and "soldiers". Interestingly too, considering that the cult of Hephaestus seemed likely to have been blacksmiths and armourers, termites are now believed to have evolved from cockroaches.

That's quite a quaint little analogy until you realise, they are one of the most successful organisms on Earth, having colonised most landmasses apart from Antarctica and are responsible for causing serious damage to buildings, and crop plantations.

You might wonder what good I can possibly find to tell you about termites.

Measuring little more than 4mm, they play a fundamental part in recycling dead trees and compost. As they tunnel, they aerate and improve the soil.

Imagine if that were true, and that the soldiers were termites, catalysed into action by the high priestess smashing a stalactite with her double axe. She would have been responsible for instructing one of the most successful civilizations the human species has ever known, and that history would remember for millennia.

Standard interpretation agrees that the Eleusinian initiation celebrated the coming of wheat and its personification, but also the journey an initiate would come to take to comprehend life and its mysteries on a deeper level. The initiate would come to understand the biological processes that created them and how to intervene with those that could threaten to destroy them. As an apprentice, now you too bear the responsibility of Earth stewardship.

If nothing else, please know the bees need *you*.

We lose more species every year, and not just bees, but so many other pollinators too. There is no doubt the problem is complex. The four main areas of concern are believed to be parasites, lack of biodiversity, cellular (mobile) technology that interferes with their ability to navigate electromagnetic fields in relation to the sun, and pesticides.

Farmers still receive no initiatives to persuade them against pesticides in this country, so every day more pollinators are found poisoned with their long proboscises hanging out.

Appallingly, in January 2021, the British government reversed its previous decision to ban neonicotinoids, allowing them to be sprayed onto sugar beet, despite the growing levels of concern, not only for bees, but also the deleterious effects sugar has on our health.

Studies show that it isn't only pollinators that neonicotinoids harm, but aquatic life suffers too, and they can actively contribute to biodiversity decline. Research suggests the chemicals weaken bees' immune systems and injure baby bees' brain development leaving them unable to fly. Another study demonstrated that honey samples are being contaminated by neonicotinoids too.

Dave Goulson is a Professor of Biology at University of Sussex specialising in bee ecology. He has published more than 300 scientific articles on the ecology and conservation of bumblebees and other insects. He warns that one teaspoon of neonic is enough to kill 1.25 billion honey bees, equivalent to four lorryloads of the insects.

We should be holding garden centres to account too. Would you believe, there are still some who place pictures of bees on their plant labels to encourage us to buy them, then spray the leaves with neonicotinoids. I felt sick to the stomach when I learnt this, feeling like an accessory after the fact. I have now become very good at propagating my own plants from seed and from cuttings.

Too many stretches of land have no flowers on them at all, so many insects die of exhaustion or thirst before they get the chance to find their way home. Please consider planting some wild flowers in unclaimed spaces along your roads. The dried out soil at the bottom of a lamppost, for example, might be the difference of life or death for your local bees. They desperately need pollen runways, and it is so easy to create them.

If you can donate a bit of your lawn or patio space for the pollinators, they'd be grateful, and don't be too tidy with the clippers. Leave mowing a bit later because dandelions are one of their biggest sources of pollen until the bramble flowers appear. Think crocuses and pussy willow in the spring and lots of asters in autumn for that last pollen feast before the cold.

Make bee baths to help them. A little water in a dish with some pebbles for them to stand on will really help. Please do not leave sugar water or honey which can give them infections.

Remember the plants that offer them resistance against their parasitic infestation. They tend to be their favourite sources of pollen too. Mint, thyme, wintergreen, and Artemisia species are all tiny bits of help on that front.

Get wise on the creatures that can kill your pollinators too. In Britain, watch out for Asian Hornets. Only a handful have been spotted so far, but we must be vigilant as they are the scourge of France's hives. Each needs to eat upwards of 50 bees a day to survive, so they are voracious predators. Nests can contain as many as 4000 of these. Just 12 hornets predating outside a hive is enough to paralyse it to death. If you think you spot them or one of their nests, call your local council or beekeeping society.

Conclusion

And so, as I write these last paragraphs, oddly, on the day that would have been the last day of the Mysteries, look how far you've come. Most assuredly, you have been initiated into some of the secrets of Eleusis and the kingdom of the bees.

But can you call yourself Bee *Mistress* now?

Can I, in fact?

Hardly.

A bee shamanism apprenticeship takes 13 years, so I have 12 more left to go.

Hopefully though, you too now know a little of what The Bee Mistress knows.

As for the strength of my pelvic floor alone, there's way more work to do. The Earth sipping meditation requires a great deal of pelvic discipline. I was excited to report that, after about three months' practice, I had finally managed to complete my six rounds of four rotations. The glee was short lived, when I found six rounds was just stage one on the journey. The Bee Mistress can do 144!

No wonder the queen bee needs attendants! I can't imagine there's any time in the day for anything else. It's a focusing thought that the Bee Mistress was considered to have mastery of the spiritual levels we now imagine for someone like the Dalai Lama.

There really aren't many definitive conclusions we can draw. I suspect every generation of women that passes might make their own assumptions about the Melissae, and each person that studies them probably overlays their story with their own ideals of what *they* perceive magical women to be. I have tried not to do so, but it is unavoidable in some respects, I think.

You and I have an advantage though because healing capabilities of *M. officinalis* have never been doubted.

Continually, the knowledge about it has never wavered. It's always been about joy, freedom from depression, an end to digestive problems and liberation from menstrual pain.

The Melissae had many skills. They were oracles, diviners, soul midwives and skilled energy practitioners. They had many tools. Sacred geometry, rituals, music, and they also had fragrance. That's never been a secret. Incense and the power of aromatic plants have always been acknowledged as access points in sacred practice. In this case though, we did a very human thing. We weren't the only species that operates in this realm. Just as *M. officinalis* has always been a gynaecological doctor, it's highly unlikely that the chemical make-up of either it, or Nasonov, has ever changed. This was the connection between two realms, the cerebral portal that allows you to enter the natural worlds, and specifically the hive. It's highly unlikely that this marker of consciousness has ever changed. Goddess willing, it never will.

The bee shamanesses were mistresses of their laboratories, influencing their energetic field with focused intention, meditation, melody, and fragrance. These energetic centres connected them to far away cosmic realms, to their internal organs but most of all to their emotional body.

I think it will be hard for our 21st century world to reintegrate the Shaman archetype into our psyches, because it no longer values depth. Each generation emerging, demands information and healing are given to them faster than the speed of light. Very few people want to go deeper any more, and the breadth of learning that is required to become a shaman is vast. But more than that, it requires a level of valour we no longer recognise or admire. We applaud the heroism of our warriors and admire the ambassadors of peace, but how many of us have the mettle to give up everything in search of the cause of *gnosis*? That deep empathy and feeling, of discovering and becoming? It takes time, dedication, unintelligible numbers of studious hours and devotion.

Have I achieved it? Have I heck! But for the first time in my life, I can start to see a path emerging of where I want to go. I can feel a tangible sense of purpose, and in that there is a deeper sense of strength and calm than I have had before.

I used the word grok at one point in the book. It's a strange word that has always rumbled around my family's vocabulary, and I was surprised when one person who has always been close to us seemed never to have heard it before. I told them it was to consider something spiritual deeply, but actually, that fell short. More, it is to understand something empathically, feel it at your core. That is very much the shamaness's route, to bestow so much devotion, so much desire to understand that eventually you can feel as someone or something else does.

And then the shapeshift can begin, not just seeing and loving the bee but having even the smallest sense of what that bee might feel. And just like that, you realise you are far from being a fully-grown woman, little more than a nymph in the cell, craving to be fed a little more bee bread, in the hope that one day soon you might emerge with wings. Who knows, maybe if you are lucky/unlucky enough to be chosen, you might even be chosen to be gorged on royal jelly.

From the Author

That you made it to this page means everything to me. Your compassion and attention to the story is touching. There is another volume to this story, the first part, the tales of the Lemon Balm herb itself and the incredible things it can do. If you have enjoyed this story, perhaps you would enjoy more of the strange instances that I ascribe to the plant rather than to the priestesses.

That book is called:

Lemon Balm *Melissa Officinalis* – The Initiation Plant of the Shamanistic Bee Priestesses and The Essential Oil of Every Day Miracles.

I hope you will want to learn more about my work with the Melissae, with Aromythology and of course essential oils in general.

If so, please head over to my website:

www.thesecrethealer.co.uk

References

1. **Kevan, Peter.** Bees Make Parsnip Seeds. [Online] https://www.researchgate.net/profile/Peter-Kevan-2/ publication/261911759_Bees_Make_Parsnip_Seeds/ links/00463535e5dbf7f61f000000/Bees-Make-Parsnip-Seeds.pdf

2. **Bertrand, Azra and Bertrand, Seren.** *Womb Awakening*. Inner Traditions/Bear & Company, Kindle Edition, 2017, p. 3.

3. *Upper Paleolithic Venus Figurines and Interpretations of Prehistoric Gender Representations.* **Vandewettering, Kaylea R.** 2015.

4. **Gimbutas, Marija.** *Civilization of the Goddess.* San Francisco: Harper, 1991.

5. **White, Randall.** The Women of Brassempouy: A Century of Research and Interpretation. 1999.

6. Venus Figurines of the Upper Paleolithic. **Nesbitt, Shawntelle.** 2001.

7. **Redmond, Layne.** *When The Drummers Were Women: A Spiritual History of Rhythm.* New York: Crown Publications, 1997.

8. Monitoring of Swarming Sounds in Bee Hives for Early Detection of the Swarming Period. **Ferrari, S.; Silva, M.; Guarino, M.; Berckmans, D.** *Computers and Electronics in Agriculture,* Volume 64, Issue 1, November 2008, pp. 72-77.

9. **Bortolotti, Laura and Costa, Cecilia.** Chemical Communication in the Honey Bee Society (Chapter 5). [Online] *Neurobiology of Chemical Communication.* 1980.

10. **Lucian.** *De Dea Syria,* vol iii., p. 382.

11. **Matteoli, Richard L.** Priapus: Prostitution, Genital Dismembering Goddesses, Sacred Penis Handshake in Horny Fertility. *Academia* [Online]. Date unlisted.

12. **Hammad, Manal B.** Bees and Beekeeping in Ancient Egypt.

Journal of Association of Arab Universities for Tourism and Hospitality, 2018.

13. **Kritsky, Gene.** *The Tears of Re.* Oxford University Press, 2015.
14. **Budge, E.A. Wallis.** *The Gods of The Egyptians.* Dover Publications, 2000.
15. **Blavatsky, Helena Petrovna & Mead, George Robert Stow.** *The Theosophical Glossary.* 1892.
16. **Bonwick, James.** *Egyptian Belief and Modern Thought.* Falcon Wings Press, 2015.
17. **Plutarch.** *Moralia.* [Online] http://penelope.uchicago. edu/Thayer/E/Roman/Texts/Plutarch/Moralia/Isis_and_ Osiris*/C.html
18. *The Mysterious Serapeum of Egypt.* https://www.youtube. com/watch?v=CxgHeh9Mlrg
19. **Rietveld, James.** *Artemis of the Ephesians.* Kindle, 2014.
20. **Correa, Katherine.** Artemis Ephesia and Sacred Bee. [Online] https://honors.adelphi.edu/wp-content/blogs. dir/741/files/2018/06/Honors-College-Symposium-Volume-XII.pdf#page=74 (2015).
21. **Whitfield, B.G.** Virgil and the Bees: A study in Ancient Apicultural Lore. *Greece & Rome*, 99-117. [Online] 7 11. http://www.jstor.org/stable/641360 (1956).
22. **Burkert, Walter.** *Greek Religion.* Cambridge, Massachusetts: Harvard University Press, 1985.
23. **Dodds, E.R.** *The Greeks and the Irrational.* University of California Press, 2nd edition, 2004.
24. **Carson, Rachel.** *The Honey Bee and Apian Imagery in Classical Literature.* University of Washington, 2015.
25. **Kealey, Alexander.** Pythagorean Shamanism. [Online] https://www.scribd.com/document/133080608/ Pythagorean-Shamanism-by-Alexander-Kealey (2017).
26. **Evangeliou, Christos.** *The Hellenistic Philosophy: Between Europe, Africa and Asia.* Institute of Global Cultural Studies, Binghampton University, 1997.

27. **Hughes, Bettany.** *Venus and Aphrodite.* Orion, Kindle Edition.

28. **Mead, George Robert Stow.** *Orpheus: Theosophy of the Greeks.* Archive.org. [Online] [Cited: 5 12 2021.] https://archive.org/stream/MeadGRSOrpheus/Mead%20GRS%20-%20Orpheus_djvu.txt

29. **Lawler, Lillian B.** Bee Dances and the "Sacred Bees". *J Stor.* [Online] 1954. [Cited: 03 12 2019.] www.jstor.org/stable/4343554

30. **Shannon, Laura.** The Cosmic Dance (Part Two) by Laura Shannon. [Online] 04 08. [Cited: 13 11 2020.] https://feminismandreligion.com/2018/08/04/the-cosmic-dance-part-two-by-laura-shannon/ (2018).

31. **Buxton, Simon.** *The Shamanic Way of the Bee.* Destiny Books, 2006, p. 115.

32. **Naylor, Jennifer.** Personal conversation. 2021.

33. **Avalon, Annwyn.** *The Way of the Water Priestess.* Red Wheel/Weiser, Kindle Edition, 2021, pp. xii-xiii.

34. **Robertson, Noel.** The Riddle of the Arrhephoria at Athens. *Harvard Studies in Classical Philology.* 1983.

35. **Pausanias.** Description of Greece 7. 19. 1-20. 1. [Online] https://www.theoi.com/Cult/ArtemisCult2.html

36. **Turner, Judy Ann.** *Hiereiai: Acquisition of Feminine Priesthoods in Ancient Greece.* PhD dissertation, University of California, Santa Barbara, 1983.

37. **Mansfield, J.M.** *The Robe of Athena and the Panathenaic Peplos.* Dissertation, Berkeley, 1985.

38. **Sédir, Paul. Translated by R. Bailey.** *Occult Botany: Sédir's Concise Guide to Magical Plants.* Rochester: Inner Traditions/Bear & Company, 2021.

39. Ancient Greek. https://en.wiktionary.org/wiki/%CE%B4%CE%AF%CE%B4%CF%89%CE%BC%CE%B9#Ancient_Greek [Online].

40. **Jung, C.G.** *Man and His Symbols*. Random House Publishing Group, 2012.
41. **Rohde.** *Psyche.* 1961, pp. 206-210.
42. **Dignas, Beate and Trampedach, Kai.** *Practitioners of the Divine: Greek Priests and Religious Officials from Homer to Heliodorus*. Hellenic Studies Series 30. Washington, DC: Center for Hellenic Studies, 2008.
43. **Worthen, T.D.** The Pleiades and Hesperides: Finding Parity with an Astronomical Key. *Elsevier Science.* [Online] https://www.sciencedirect.com/sdfe/pdf/download/eid/1-s2.0-0083665695000097/first-page-pdf (1995).
44. **Morgado, Kim.** The Honey Bear. Bee Mythology. [Online] [Cited: 25 02 2021.] http://www.thehoneybear.co.za/bee-mythology.htm (Date unlisted).
45. **Szymanski, Christine.** Artemis. [Online] https://www.facebook.com/BridgeToLemuriaFindingYourWayHome/photos/the-bee-is-more-honored-than-other-animals-not-because-she-labors-but-because-sh/365235150237546/
46. **Riley, Lucinda.** Myths and Legends. [Online] [Cited: 25 02 2021.] http://lucindariley.co.uk/myths-and-legends/ (2018).
47. **Daily Sabah.** Six statues unearthed at Magnesia on the Meander. [Online] [Cited: 27 02 2021.] https://www.dailysabah.com/history/2018/07/28/six-2000-year-old-greek-statues-discovered-in-southwestern-turkey (2018).
48. **Smith, William.** *A Dictionary of Greek and Roman Biography, Mythology and Geography, Volume 2*. John Murray, 1890.
49. **Pindar.** *Pythian 4.* 60.
50. **Cyrino, Monica S.** *Aphrodite* (Gods and Heroes of the Ancient World). New York and London: Routledge, 2010.
51. **Johnson, David.** Cypriot picrolite cruciform figure: Middle Chalcolithic 3000 - 2700 BC. [Online] [Cited: 03 1 2020.] https://ant.david-johnson.co.uk/catalogue/65

52. **Liddell, Henry George and Scott, Robert.** *A Greek-English Lexicon.* Perseus Project, 1843.

53. **Encyclopaedia Britannica.** Aphrodite. [Online] https://www.britannica.com/topic/Aphrodite-Greek-mythology

54. **Daly, Ariella.** Conversation during Melissa training [Online].

55. **Glenn, Lori.** Personal correspondence.

56. **Athenogorus.** *Legatio,* vol. ii., p. 179.

57. **Ovid.** *Opera,* vol. iii., Fasti, lib. iv. ll. 219, 220.

58. **Hislop, Rev. Alexander.** *The Two Babylons, Or The Papal Worship Proved to Be The Worship of Nimrod and His Wife.* 1862.

59. **Ampelius, Lucius.** *I Libro ad Maccrinum apud.* Bryant Volume 3, p. 161, 3rd Century.

60. **Hwang, Deok-Sang; Kim, Sun Kwang; and Bae, Hyunsu.** Therapeutic Effects of Bee Venom on Immunological and Neurological Diseases. [Online] 2015. https://www.ncbi.nlm.nih.gov/pmc/articles/PMC4516920/

61. **Chrystal, Paul.** *In Bed With The Greeks.* Amberley Books, 2016.

62. **Misy.** Mindat.org. [Online] https://www.mindat.org/min-6126.html

63. **Halperin, David.** *A Hundred Years of Homosexuality.* Routledge, 1990.

64. **Pindar.** Pythian Ode. 3.5.

65. **Capaldi, E.A., Dyer, F.C.** The role of orientation flights on homing performance in honeybees. *Journal of Experimental Biology,* 1999. [Online] https://journals.biologists.com/jeb/article/202/12/1655/8025/The-role-of-orientation-flights-on-homing

66. **Winston, Mark L.** *The Biology of The Honeybee.* Harvard, 1991.

67. **Johnson, Brian.** Global information sampling in the honey bee. [Online] 2008. https://pubmed.ncbi.nlm.nih.gov/18330538/

68. *Studies in Folk Life: Essays in Honour of Iorwerth C. Peate* (RLE Folklore). **Geraint Jenkins** (ed.). Taylor and Francis, 2015.

69. **Homer.** *Odyssey.* Book 11, pp. 71-74.

70. **Agelarakis, Anagnostis P.** Arcane Whispers Echoed from Monumental Tomb "M" at Orthi Petra in Eleutherna. *Adelphi University Anthropology Faculty Publications,* 2012.

71. **Dieu-Le-Veut, Annie.** *The Sacred Sex Rites of Ishtar: Shamanic sexual healing and sex magic.* The Holistic Works, Kindle Edition, 2015.

72. [Online] https://www.nairaland.com/3830673/shocking-story-ugandan-woman-gives

73. [Online] https://gnnliberia.com/2020/05/28/in-uganda-woman-claims-she-gave-birth-to-a-snake/

74. [Online] https://www.hellenion.org/festivals/skiraphoria/

75. **van Die, Diana; Burger, Henry G.; Teede, Helena J.; Bone, Kerry M.** Vitex agnus-castus extracts for female reproductive disorders: a systematic review of clinical trials. [Online] https://pubmed.ncbi.nlm.nih.gov/23136064/. *Planta Medica,* 2013.

76. **Versnel, H.S.** The Festival for Bona Dea and The Thesmophoria. *Greece and Rome,* Volume xxxix. https://www.jstor.org/stable/643119#. Volume 1, 1992.

77. **Hamilton, E.** *The Greek Way.* W.W. Norton and Company, 1930.

78. **Taylor, Thomas.** *The Eleusinian and Bacchic Mysteries: A Dissertation.* [Online] 23 12 1891.

79. **Butler, Samuel.** Ὅμηρος Ἰλιάς *(The Iliad).* 1.513 (456), 1898.

80. **Cicero.** *Laws.* II, xiv, 36.

81. **You Go Culture** Virtual Tour - Eleusinia - The Sacred Way - Hiera Odos. [Online] http://yougoculture.com/virtual-tour/eleusina/myth/the-sacred-way-hiera-odos#:~:text=The%20ancient%20road%20connecting%20Athens,plain%20connected%20Attica%20with%20Peloponnesus

82. **Shannon, Laura.** Women's Ritual Dances: An Ancient Source of Healing. In *Dancing on the Earth: Women's Stories of Healing Through Dance*. Findhorn Press, 2011.

83. **Wright, Dudley.** *The Eleusinian Mysteries and Rites.* Theosophical Publishing House, Project Gutenberg, www. gutenberg.net (1919).

84. **Freeman, Jacqueline.** *Song of Increase.* [Online] Sounds True, Kindle Edition, 2016.

85. **Burkert, W.** Plutarch, fragment 168, found in *Gifts to the Gods: Offerings in Perspective: Surrender, Distribution, Exchange*, T. Linders and G. Nordquist (eds.). Upsalla, 1987.

86. **Baranitharan et al.** Chemical composition and laboratory investigation of Melissa officinalis essential oil against human malarial vector mosquito, Anopheles stephensi L. (Diptera: Culicidae). *Phytochemistry and Entomotoxicity*, 2016. https:// www.researchgate.net/publication/311776069_Chemical_ composition_and_laboratory_investigation_of_Melissa_ officinalis_essential_oil_against_human_malarial_vector_ mosquito_Anopheles_stephensi_L_Diptera_Culicidae

87. **Martins, Thércia Gabrielle Teixeira et al.** Larvicidal activity of microparticles of Melissa officinalis L. essential oil (Lamiaceae) against Aedes aegypti (Diptera, Culicidae). https://www.researchgate.net/publication/348581670_ Larvicidal_activity_of_microparticles_of_Melissa_ officinalis_L_essential_oil_Lamiaceae_against_Aedes_ aegypti_Diptera_Culicidae (2021).

88. **Dell'Amore, Christine.** Dung Beetles Navigate Via the Milky Way, First Known in Animal Kingdom. *National Geographic*. [Online] [Cited: 09 10 2021.] https://www. nationalgeographic.com/animals/article/dung-beetles-milky-way-navigation (23 January 2013).

89. **Gardner, A., Ross, L.** The evolution of hermaphroditism by an infectious male-derived cell lineage: an inclusive-fitness analysis. *American Naturalist*, 2011.

About the Author

Elizabeth Ashley is an international speaker for the International Federation of Aromatherapists and the UK Director for the National Association of Holistic Aromatherapists. She is a prolific writer of professional articles, having written for the IFA magazine *Aromatherapy Thymes*, *Aromatika* (Hungarian and English), *In Essence*, *Aromatica* (Australian), the NAHA *Journal* and *Holistic Therapist Magazine*. She qualified as an aromatherapist in 1993, and then passed her Advanced Aromatherapy Diploma in 1994. She has been practising aromatherapy for almost 30 years.

In 1999, she fell into a whole new career in the aggressive commercial sector of recruitment consultancy. There she discovered her father's second-hand car salesman genes had passed along and found she had quite a gift of the gab! More than that, she discovered she could sell... and then some.

In 2008, Elizabeth fell ill during pregnancy with a blood clot in her lungs. The pulmonary embolism prevented her from working on the telephone, and so she started to write. Very quickly she gained her first contract as a ghostwriter... a recipe book for cheesecakes! Her aromatherapy writing career culminated with her writing seven Amazon category number one best-sellers for other people, until her family and friends interceded and encouraged The Secret Healer to step out of the shadow. She has self-published 20 aromatherapy books in her own name, of which 12 have also become Amazon category number one best-sellers.

Many of her books are aimed at helping qualified aromatherapists to expand their healing repertoire and build their businesses. She also writes for people who have an interest in essential oils and want to learn how to heal. Her in-depth essential oil profiles chart the healing properties of plants from the most arcane depths of historic folklore up to the scientific lab trials of today. She has presented her work at professional conferences in the US, China, Hungary, and Bulgaria and her work has been translated into Hungarian and Portuguese.

In 2018, she co-hosted The Beyond The Essential Oil Recipe Summit with Hungarian aromatherapist Gergely Hollodi. The hugely successful event was the first ever online summit for professional aromatherapists.

Her fascination with the Lemon Balm plant began in 2018, which led her to discover bee priestesses practices. She has been training as a Melissa bee priestess and a beekeeper. This encouraged her to develop her own modality of aromatherapy. Aromythology is inhalation of essential oils with ancient Greek contemplations, based on the idea that the priestess devours fragrance like a bee.

She lives in Shropshire with her husband and youngest son, kept company by their bees, Staffordshire Bull Terrier, Bella, and many shoals of tropical fish! Her elder son and daughter are now grown and have flown the nest and make her prouder than anything ever could. Elizabeth Ashley is The Secret Healer.

Other Books By Elizabeth Ashley

The Complete Guide to Clinical Aromatherapy &
Essential Oils for the Physical Body
ASIN: B00PM7PB2I

Essential Oils for the Mind Body Spirit: The Holistic
Medicine of Clinical Aromatherapy
ASIN: B00Q1G3SZG

The Essential Oil Liver Cleanse: The Professional
Aromatherapist's Liver Detox
ASIN: B00PKARDBO

The Professional Stress Solution: Essential Oils,
Aromatherapy and Holistic Healing Stress Management
Techniques for The Professional Aromatherapist
ASIN: B00PR304CE

The Aromatherapy Eczema Treatment: The Professional
Aromatherapist's Guide to Healing Eczema, Itchy Skin Rashes
and Atopic Dermatitis with Essential Oils and
Holistic Medicine
ASIN: B00PKD0N9K

The Aromatherapy Bronchitis Treatment: Support the
Respiratory System with Essential Oils and Holistic
Medicine for COPD, Emphysema, Acute and
Chronic Bronchitis Symptoms.
ASIN: B00T0BJ74U

Monarda: A Native American Medicine: How To Meditate
And Heal The Physical Body Using Medicinal Plants and
Essential Oils For The Mind Body Spirit
ASIN: B00U3R6GCG

Vetiver: An Ayurvedic Medicine: How To Meditate And
Heal The Physical Body Using Medicinal Plants and
Essential Oils For The Mind Body Spirit
ASIN: B00U4F0C72

Rose: Goddess Medicine: The Timeless Elixir of Ancient Egypt,
Ayurveda, Chinese Medicine, Essential Oils and
Modern Medicine
ASIN: B00YG0JYB6

Clary Sage: Salvia Sclarea: Natural Estrogen?: Alleviate
Symptoms of Menopause, Premenstrual Syndrome and Period
Pains. Reduce Muscle Cramps and Restless Leg Syndrome.
ASIN: B018KIYK6I

Sweet Basil: Ocimum Basilicum – The Essential Oil of
Empowerment: How To Heal The Mind Body Spirit Using
Medicinal Plants And Aromatherapy
ASIN: B012J0GPS4

Holy Basil – Ayurvedic Medicine's Tulsi: How To Meditate
And Heal The Physical Body Using Medicinal Plants and
Essential Oils For The Mind Body Spirit
ASIN: B00VHR8IWW

Spikenard - A Woman Anoints Jesus's feet - Did She Use the Spikenard of Aromatherapy? Nardostachys jatamansi – An Essential Oil And Medicinal Plant for Digestive Problems, Nervous Disorders, Anxiety, Insomnia, Epilepsy, Seizures and Fear.
ASIN: B01D19L17M

Helichrysum For The Wound That Will Not Heal: The Lost History of Immortelle, The Everlasting Flower, Its Chemistry and Helichrysum Italicum Essential Oil Uses in Aromatherapy.
ASIN: B01M5AH4PA

Cannabis: High CBD Hemp, Hemp Essential Oil and Hemp Seed Oil: The Cannabis Medicines of Aromatherapy's Own Medical Marijuana
ASIN: B074LW4C4M

Sales Strategies for Gentle Souls: Targeted Sales Training for Professional Aromatherapists
ASIN: B00PIYDYBU

And

Lemon Balm **Melissa Officinalis** *– The Initiation Plant of the Shamanistic Bee Priestesses and The Essential Oil of Every Day Miracles*
Not yet published – ISBN to follow

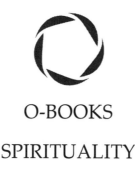

O-BOOKS

SPIRITUALITY

O is a symbol of the world, of oneness and unity; this eye represents knowledge and insight. We publish titles on general spirituality and living a spiritual life. We aim to inform and help you on your own journey in this life.

If you have enjoyed this book, why not tell other readers by posting a review on your preferred book site?

Recent bestsellers from O-Books are:

Heart of Tantric Sex
Diana Richardson
Revealing Eastern secrets of deep love and intimacy to Western couples.
Paperback: 978-1-90381-637-0 ebook: 978-1-84694-637-0

Crystal Prescriptions
The A-Z guide to over 1,200 symptoms and their healing crystals
Judy Hall
The first in the popular series of eight books, this handy little guide is packed as tight as a pill-bottle with crystal remedies for ailments.
Paperback: 978-1-90504-740-6 ebook: 978-1-84694-629-5

Take Me To Truth
Undoing the Ego
Nouk Sanchez, Tomas Vieira
The best-selling step-by-step book on shedding the Ego, using the
teachings of *A Course In Miracles*.
Paperback: 978-1-84694-050-7 ebook: 978-1-84694-654-7

The 7 Myths about Love...Actually!
The Journey from your HEAD to the HEART of your SOUL
Mike George
Smashes all the myths about LOVE.
Paperback: 978-1-84694-288-4 ebook: 978-1-84694-682-0

The Holy Spirit's Interpretation of the New Testament
A Course in Understanding and Acceptance
Regina Dawn Akers
Following on from the strength of *A Course In Miracles*, NTI
teaches us how to experience the love and oneness of God.
Paperback: 978-1-84694-085-9 ebook: 978-1-78099-083-5

The Message of A Course In Miracles
A translation of the Text in plain language
Elizabeth A. Cronkhite
A translation of *A Course In Miracles* into plain, everyday
language for anyone seeking inner peace. The companion
volume, *Practicing A Course In Miracles*, offers practical lessons
and mentoring.
Paperback: 978-1-84694-319-5 ebook: 978-1-84694-642-4

Your Simple Path
Find Happiness in every step
Ian Tucker
A guide to helping us reconnect with what is really important in
our lives.
Paperback: 978-1-78279-349-6 ebook: 978-1-78279-348-9

365 Days of Wisdom
Daily Messages To Inspire You Through The Year
Dadi Janki
Daily messages which cool the mind, warm the heart and guide
you along your journey.
Paperback: 978-1-84694-863-3 ebook: 978-1-84694-864-0

Body of Wisdom
Women's Spiritual Power and How it Serves
Hilary Hart
Bringing together the dreams and experiences of women across
the world with today's most visionary spiritual teachers.
Paperback: 978-1-78099-696-7 ebook: 978-1-78099-695-0

Dying to Be Free
From Enforced Secrecy to Near Death to True Transformation
Hannah Robinson
After an unexpected accident and near-death experience, Hannah
Robinson found herself radically transforming her life, while a
remarkable new insight altered her relationship with her father, a
practising Catholic priest.
Paperback: 978-1-78535-254-6 ebook: 978-1-78535-255-3

The Ecology of the Soul
A Manual of Peace, Power and Personal Growth for Real People
in the Real World
Aidan Walker
Balance your own inner Ecology of the Soul to regain your
natural state of peace, power and wellbeing.
Paperback: 978-1-78279-850-7 ebook: 978-1-78279-849-1

Not I, Not other than I
The Life and Teachings of Russel Williams
Steve Taylor, Russel Williams
The miraculous life and inspiring teachings of one of the World's
greatest living Sages.
Paperback: 978-1-78279-729-6 ebook: 978-1-78279-728-9

On the Other Side of Love
A woman's unconventional journey towards wisdom
Muriel Maufroy
When life has lost all meaning, what do you do?
Paperback: 978-1-78535-281-2 ebook: 978-1-78535-282-9

Practicing A Course In Miracles
A translation of the Workbook in plain language, with
mentor's notes
Elizabeth A. Cronkhite
The practical second and third volumes of The Plain-Language
A Course In Miracles.
Paperback: 978-1-84694-403-1 ebook: 978-1-78099-072-9

Quantum Bliss
The Quantum Mechanics of Happiness, Abundance, and Health
George S. Mentz
Quantum Bliss is the breakthrough summary of success and spirituality secrets that customers have been waiting for.
Paperback: 978-1-78535-203-4 ebook: 978-1-78535-204-1

The Upside Down Mountain
Mags MacKean
A must-read for anyone weary of chasing success and happiness – one woman's inspirational journey swapping the uphill slog for the downhill slope.
Paperback: 978-1-78535-171-6 ebook: 978-1-78535-172-3

Your Personal Tuning Fork
The Endocrine System
Deborah Bates
Discover your body's health secret, the endocrine system, and 'twang' your way to sustainable health!
Paperback: 978-1-84694-503-8 ebook: 978-1-78099-697-4

Readers of ebooks can buy or view any of these bestsellers by clicking on the live link in the title. Most titles are published in paperback and as an ebook. Paperbacks are available in traditional bookshops. Both print and ebook formats are available online.
Find more titles and sign up to our readers' newsletter at http://www.johnhuntpublishing.com/mind-body-spirit
Follow us on Facebook at https://www.facebook.com/OBooks/ and Twitter at https://twitter.com/obooks